RETURN
TO
BEAUTY

RETURN
TO
BEAUTY

OLD-WORLD RECIPES
FOR GREAT RADIANT SKIN

NARINE NIKOGOSIAN

PHOTOGRAPHS BY JUSTIN LEE WHEELER

ATRIA BOOKS

New York   London   Toronto   Sydney

This publication contains the opinions and ideas of its author. It is intended to provide helpful and informative material on the subjects addressed in the publication. It is sold with the understanding that the author and publisher are not engaged in rendering medical, health, or any other kind of personal professional services in the book. The reader should consult his or her medical, health, or other competent professional before adopting any of the suggestions in this book or drawing inferences from it.

The author and publisher specifically disclaim all responsibility for any liability, loss or risk, personal or otherwise, which is incurred as a consequence, directly or indirectly, of the use and application of any of the contents of this book.

ATRIA BOOKS

A Division of Simon & Schuster, Inc.
1230 Avenue of the Americas
New York, NY 10020

Copyright © 2009 by Narine Nikogosian

All rights reserved, including the right to reproduce this book or portions thereof in any form whatsoever. For information address Atria Books Subsidiary Rights Department, 1230 Avenue of the Americas, New York, NY 10020

First Atria Books hardcover edition November 2009

ATRIA BOOKS and colophon are trademarks of Simon & Schuster, Inc.

For information about special discounts for bulk purchases,
please contact Simon & Schuster Special Sales at
1-866-506-1949 or business@simonandschuster.com.

The Simon & Schuster Speakers Bureau can bring authors
to your live event. For more information or to book an event,
contact the Simon & Schuster Speakers Bureau at
1-866-248-3049 or visit our website at www.simonspeakers.com.

Designed by Nancy Singer

Manufactured in the United States of America

10   9   8   7   6   5   4   3   2

Library of Congress Cataloging in Publication Data

Nikogosian, Narine.
    Return to beauty: old-world recipes for great radiant skin / Narine Nikogosian.
        p. cm.
    1. Skin care and hygiene. I. Title.
    RL87.N55   2009
    646.7'2—dc22   2009998147

ISBN 978-1-4391-2606-6
ISBN 978-1-4391-6817-2 (ebook)

This book is dedicated to you, the reader.

May it take you home to your own beauty;

you will find it in your heart.

Contents

RETURN
TO
BEAUTY

INTRODUCTION

The truth about real beauty is that it's up to each person to bring it out from within—by the words we think and use, the foods we eat, and how we take care of the world around us. I grew up in Armenia, where fresh fruit and vegetable stands overflowed on every corner—ripe with delicious scents and brilliant colors. In Armenia, we didn't just eat the fruit, we used the fruit—even to create skin care products. Today, beauty is a $50 billion-a-year industry. The modern woman uses products that can be expensive and, worse, often contain toxins. For example, a top-selling skin care line currently on the market that can be purchased at any grocery store in the country contains (according to the Environmental Working Group) an ingredient so toxic that it has been banned in Canada and by the European Union. How does this make you beautiful?

The use of fresh foods to create a healthy beauty regimen has thrived since ancient times. Cleopatra took milk baths. I hail from a long line of women seriously interested in skin care. During World War II, the Russian government gave each citizen a daily ration of one piece of bread and a pat of butter. That was all the people had to eat for an entire day. My grandmother ate the bread but spread the butter on her face as a moisturizer. That's old-world wisdom. That's a determined woman!

Old-world wisdom for skin care offers different recipes depending upon each person's skin type. For instance, if you have very dry skin, in the winter your moisturizer would be completely different from that of a woman with oily skin. A woman with oily skin can add lemon juice to almost any recipe; however, a woman with dry skin needs soothing foods like avocados to stay hydrated.

I began to learn the secrets to having beautiful, healthy skin when I was a little girl. I would beg to go with my grandmother and mother to the local salon where they received their facials. Watching the beautiful aesthetician's hands dance across my mother's face, I would memorize the movements to practice later in front of the mirror in my room back at home. I started experimenting with whatever foods were in our kitchen (vegetables, fruits, grains, and dairy), creating various concoctions that I would try on my own face. Some recipes were successful; others felt like glue.

As I grew older, I experimented with my new knowledge, adding to it my love of astrology. I created recipes based upon the various needs of each sun sign. I then invited my friends over to try my treatments. Through trial and error, I became successful at treating all different types of skin conditions.

I can't wait to go to work each morning. I'm the luckiest woman in the world.

A NOTE TO THE READER

Welcome, new friends!

To create the happiest and most successful journey for you, this book has been broken down into three main sections: Seasons, Sun Signs, and Simple Solutions.

The first section, Seasons, contains recipes for each skin type for every season. These recipes should be used as your daily skin care regimen throughout the year. The recipes in the second section, Sun Signs, are intended to be playful and enhance your overall experience. For common concerns, please refer to the Simple Solutions section. There you will find quick remedies for everything from dark under-eye circles and pimples to brittle nails and split ends.

In the fourth section, you'll find recipes to follow if you're pregnant. These recipes focus on remedies for the unique challenges you're faced with during this happy time.

When you can't afford a professional facial or your day calendar is full, I've provided some beauty secrets with easy-to-follow steps in the section How to Give Yourself a Facial.

Last, for the man in your life, turn to the No Frills for Men pages. There you will find basic skin care recipes that even he will want to follow.

I have tried to take into account budgetary concerns as well as busy daily schedules. Most recipes are easy to make and require only ten minutes of preparation. If you don't own a food processor, use a blender. If you don't own a blender, use a mixer. If you don't own a mixer, use a potato masher. (Remember how my grandmother used the butter on her face during World War II—be creative!) If you can't afford organic, be sure to purchase fresh ingredients. If something is out of season in the region where you live, buy fresh-frozen fruit with no added sugars.

You will notice that many of my recipes contain one of these three ingredients: honey, eggs, or dairy. These healing foods make a creamy base for any cleanser or moisturizer. When heating honey or milk, remember that you want to warm it only slightly to mix it with other ingredients. Always test for temperature before using any recipe on your skin.

Most recipes are to be made the day that you intend to use them. Please remember that there are no preservatives in fresh foods, so if you double a recipe, it may not last. Always refrigerate leftovers in a clean plastic container.

Before using a recipe on your face, dab a small amount on your wrist. If your skin has an adverse reaction, discontinue usage. There are plenty of other recipes to try. Find the ones that make you feel, and look, your best.

Thank you for allowing me to share my skin care passion with you.

WHAT'S YOUR SKIN TYPE?

It's easy to determine your skin type by choosing from the definitions below.

THE SHINE FACTOR

The shine factor relates to oily and normal-to-oily skin.

OILY skin is shiny all over, all day long.

NORMAL-TO-OILY skin is shiny only in the T-zone (forehead, nose, and chin), and only at certain times of the day.

THE COMFORTABILITY FACTOR

The comfortability factor relates to dry and normal-to-dry skin.

DRY skin feels dehydrated throughout the day. In the morning, your skin feels especially tight across the cheek area.

NORMAL-TO-DRY skin feels tight and dehydrated only at certain times of the day.

MY BEAUTIFUL FACE MANTRA

Real beauty springs forth from within. Every morning before you begin your regimen, I want you to look in the mirror and repeat several times:

I AM SO BEAUTIFUL.

When you are unhappy with your appearance, don't be unkind to yourself. That's the fastest way to age. Be proactive. Take good care of your skin by giving it healthy, fresh fruits and vegetables. Keep it clean and neat. Remember to check your muscles for tension. If you find any, relax your face!

Smile! You are beautiful!

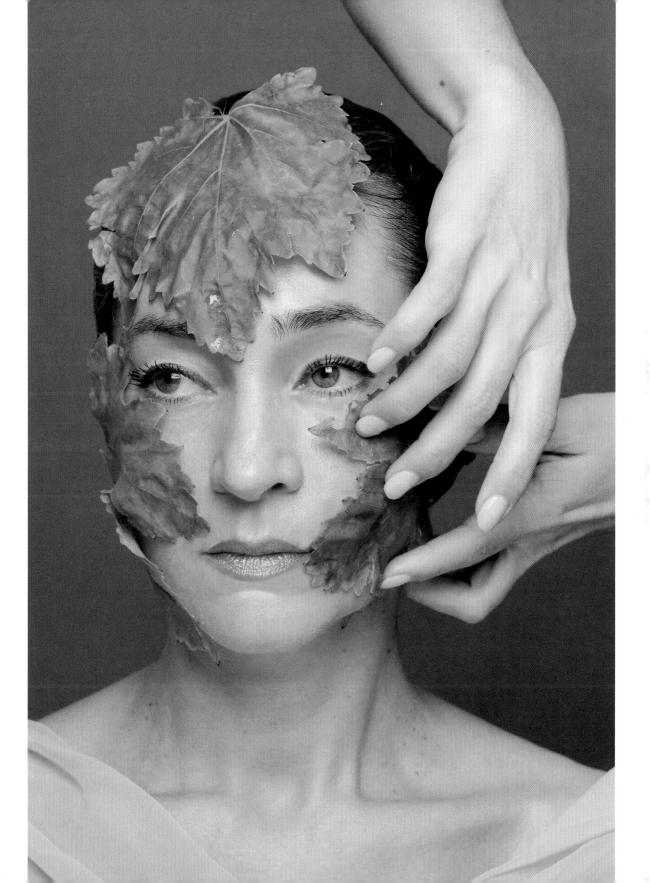

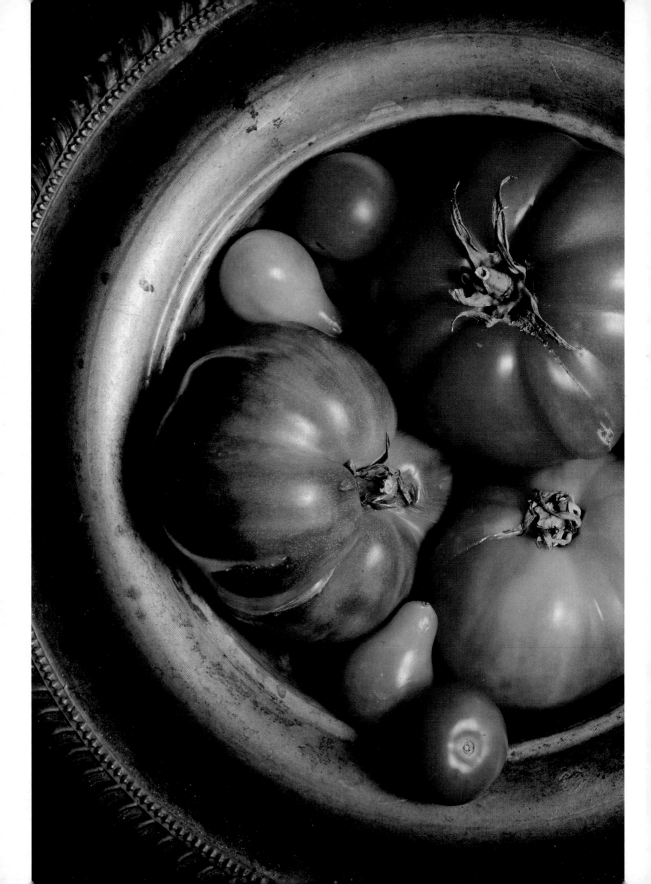

Part 1

SEASONS

Winter, spring, summer, fall—your skin has different needs for them all.

Every season comes with its own set of unique challenges. For instance, hot, humid summers can cause breakouts for those with oily skin. Women with dry skin suffer the most during colder weather.

This section provides a simple daily facial regimen for each season, based upon your skin type. The recipes are simple and economical. They will offer you beautiful results—for the rest of your life!

Before we begin, I offer a gentle reminder. Sunscreen is one of the most important things you can do for your skin in any season. I don't have a recipe for sunscreen. You must purchase one that you like. And please—remember to use it on a daily basis.

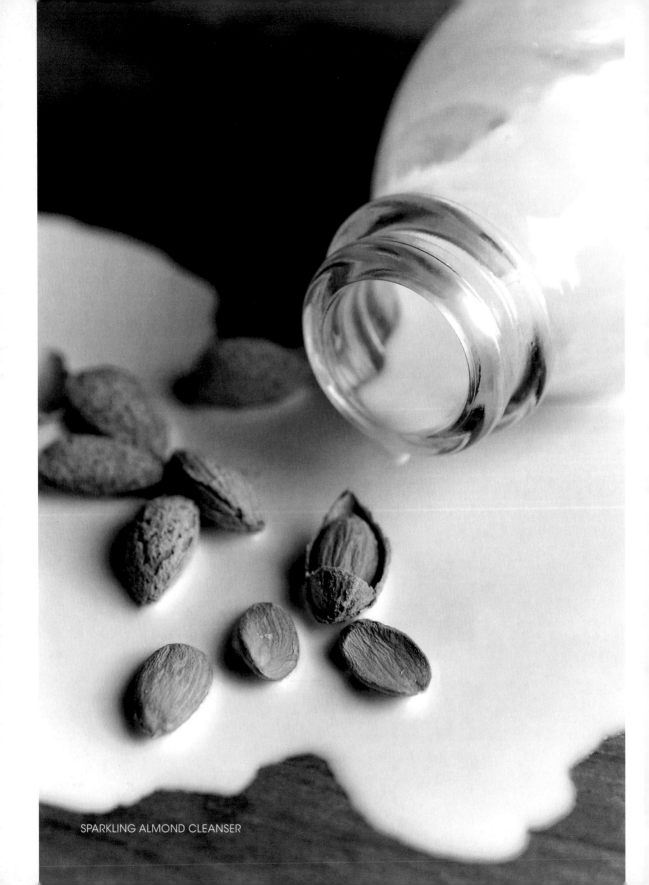

SPARKLING ALMOND CLEANSER

WINTER DRY SKIN

If you have dry skin, the cold winter months can take their toll. Fine lines appear more noticeable. Makeup application seems difficult. Your skin is dehydrated, resulting in a lifeless and flaky surface. These concerns are due to the slowing down of oil-gland production and your skin's inability to retain moisture.

My great-grandmother used fresh snow from the windowsill as a hydrating facial mask. With today's air pollution, I wouldn't recommend that technique! Almond milk, coconut oil, and olive oil are all wonderful foods for winter restoration.

Please note: In the winter, people with dry skin should not use a toner.

SHINY LEMON CLEANSER

Lemon helps your skin maintain a healthy pH balance. Sour cream contains lactic acid, which gently exfoliates. Olive oil is hydrating.

1 tablespoon lemon juice

¼ cup sour cream

1 tablespoon olive oil

PREPARATION In a small bowl, combine the lemon juice, sour cream, and oil. Mix well.

APPLICATION Wash your face and neck with this cleanser only at night. Rinse off with warm water. In the morning, splash your face and neck with cold water.

SPARKLING ALMOND CLEANSER

Almond milk is high in vitamin E and offers skin-softening properties. Honey is hydrating and gently exfoliates. Mineral water is like a party for your face.

2 tablespoons almond milk

1 teaspoon honey

¼ cup mineral water

PREPARATION In a small bowl, combine the almond milk and honey. Add the mineral water and mix well.

APPLICATION Wash your face and neck with this cleanser only at night. Rinse off with warm water. In the morning, splash your face and neck with cold water.

PRETTY FLOWERS MOISTURIZER

This is calming, soothing, and hydrating; lilies and lavender are a treat for your skin.

1 tablespoon chopped fresh lily

1 tablespoon lavender (fresh or dried)

1 teaspoon unsalted butter

1 teaspoon olive oil

1 teaspoon witch hazel

PREPARATION In a small saucepan, bring the lily and lavender to a boil in 1 cup of water. Steep for 10 minutes, then strain to remove any stems and seeds. In a blender, combine the flower liquid, butter, oil, and witch hazel. Mix well.

APPLICATION Massage a small amount over your face. Splash with warm water and pat dry.

COCO-CREAMY GREEN MOISTURIZER

Avocado is rich in vitamins A, D, and E and minerals. Coconut oil softens and protects. This is the perfect antiwrinkle, healing cure for dry skin.

¼ avocado

½ teaspoon plain yogurt

1 teaspoon lemon juice

1 teaspoon coconut oil

PREPARATION Scoop out the avocado and mash it in a bowl. Add the yogurt, lemon juice, and oil. Mix well.

APPLICATION Massage a small amount over your face.

OOH-LA-LA COCOA BUTTER EYE CREAM

Dry skin under the eye always needs extra conditioning. Cocoa butter is a great emollient. It smoothes wrinkles, leaving your skin flexible and well moisturized.

3 vitamin E capsules

2 teaspoons cocoa butter

PREPARATION Cut off the tips of the capsules. In a small bowl, combine the oil from the capsules with the cocoa butter. Mix well.

APPLICATION Gently apply around the eye area in the morning and the evening.

SPARKLING SPA HONEY SCRUB

Sugar is a gentle scrub for dry skin. Mineral-rich water combines with it to make this the perfect spalike winter facial.

1 teaspoon sugar

1 tablespoon honey

1 tablespoon mineral water

PREPARATION In a small bowl, combine the sugar and honey. Add the mineral water and mix well.

APPLICATION Using your fingers, gently scrub your face with this for 2 to 3 minutes. Rinse off with warm water. You can use this scrub in the shower.

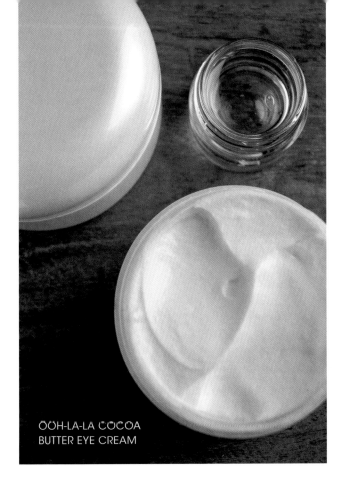

OOH-LA-LA COCOA
BUTTER EYE CREAM

SELF-HEATING COGNAC MASK

Cognac tightens pores and stimulates blood flow. Honey and cottage cheese gently exfoliate dead skin cells. The egg yolk leaves your skin soft.

1 egg yolk

1 tablespoon cottage cheese

1 teaspoon honey

1 teaspoon Cognac

PREPARATION Mix together the egg yolk and cottage cheese. Add the honey, then stir in the Cognac slowly.

APPLICATION Cover your face and neck with this mask and relax for 20 minutes. Rinse off with warm water, then apply your moisturizer.

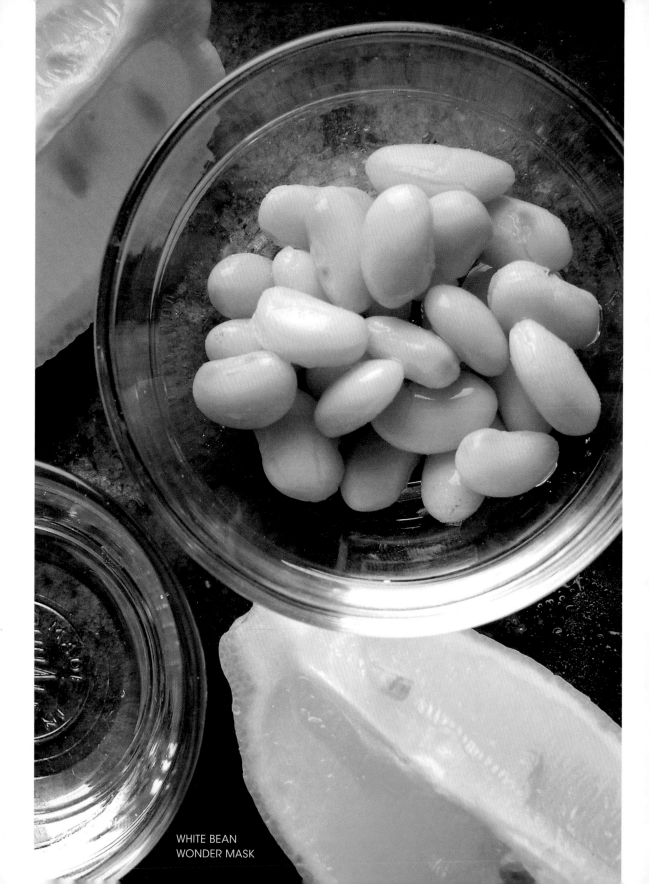

WHITE BEAN
WONDER MASK

WINTER NORMAL-TO-DRY SKIN

Whether you've been outside building a snowman or shoveling the sidewalk, cold weather can wreak havoc on tender skin. Even snow bunnies nursing hot cocoa in the lodge can fall prey to the elements!

For this reason, your winter regimen includes calming pears, soothing dairy, and a wonder food—white beans.

PEAR AND MILK CALMING CLEANSER

Pears have abundant levels of vitamins C and K, which aid in healing bruises and dark circles.

1 small ripe pear

½ cup milk

½ tablespoon sunflower oil

PREPARATION Wash the skin of the pear well, then cut it in half and remove the seeds. In a small saucepan, boil the pear halves for 5 to 7 minutes, then pat dry. In a blender, combine the pear, milk, and oil. Blend until creamy.

APPLICATION Wash your face and neck with this cleanser only at night. Rinse off with warm water. In the morning, splash your face and neck with cold water.

SWEETIE-PIE CLEANSER

Apple juice contains malic acid, which is an excellent exfoliator. Heavy cream is hydrating. The flour binds the ingredients.

3 tablespoons apple juice

1 tablespoon heavy cream

1 teaspoon flour

PREPARATION In a small bowl, mix together the apple juice and cream. Slowly stir in the flour to thicken.

APPLICATION Wash your face and neck with this cleanser only at night. Rinse off with warm water. In the morning, splash your face and neck with cold water.

CUTE DILL TONER

Dill is not only good for curing bad breath, when combined with cucumber, it makes the perfect face toner. Witch hazel naturally closes pores.

2 tablespoons chopped dill

½ cucumber

½ cup witch hazel

PREPARATION In a blender, combine the dill, cucumber, and witch hazel. Blend well, then strain.

APPLICATION Smooth this over your face using a clean cotton ball.

YUMMY YOGURT COCOA EYE CREAM

Cocoa butter is a great emollient. It will keep the thin skin around your eyes moisturized and flexible.

1 teaspoon cocoa butter

½ teaspoon plain yogurt

PREPARATION In a small saucepan, warm the cocoa butter over low heat. In a small bowl, combine the cocoa butter and yogurt. Mix well. Allow to cool before using.

APPLICATION Apply this around the eye area every morning and evening.

DREAMY CARROT MOISTURIZER

Carrots contain all the great vitamins and minerals your skin needs to stay healthy and beautiful.

1 carrot, chopped into small pieces

1 tablespoon plain yogurt

1 teaspoon sour cream

PREPARATION In a small saucepan, boil the carrot pieces for 5 to 7 minutes, then pat dry. In a small bowl, mash the carrot. Allow it to cool, then add the yogurt and sour cream for a thick consistency.

APPLICATION Apply this to your face every morning and evening after cleansing.

BEE SWEET MOISTURIZER

Hydrating and softening, these three ingredients will leave your skin baby soft.

1 teaspoon honey

1 teaspoon almond oil

½ egg yolk

PREPARATION In a small bowl, mix the ingredients together.

APPLICATION Apply to your face every morning and evening after cleansing. Splash with warm water and pat dry.

WHITE BEAN WONDER MASK

White beans are a wonder! They contain calcium, potassium, and folate. With a little bit of olive oil and lemon juice, this mask is a nutrient-rich treat!

¼ cup white beans

1 teaspoon olive oil

1 tablespoon lemon juice

PREPARATION Soak the beans overnight. In a small saucepan, bring the beans and 3 cups of water to a boil. Simmer until soft. Drain the beans. In a small bowl, mash the beans with a fork, then add the oil and lemon juice.

APPLICATION Liberally cover your face and neck with this mask and relax for 20 to 30 minutes. Rinse off with warm water, then apply your moisturizer.

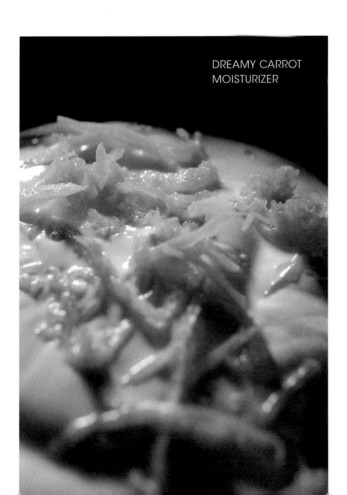

DREAMY CARROT MOISTURIZER

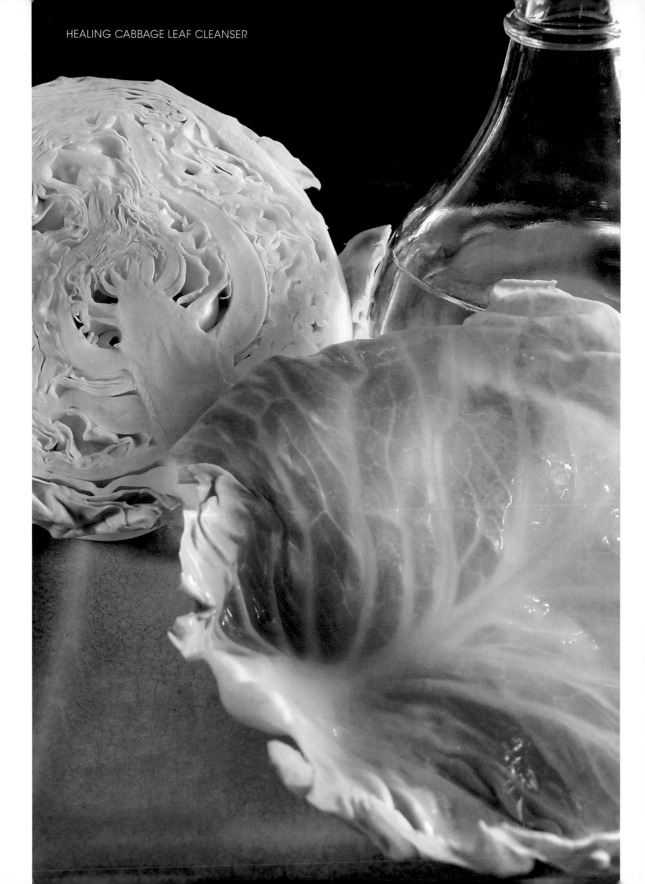

WINTER NORMAL-TO-OILY SKIN

In the old days, women stored food in cellars for sustenance during the long, dark season. Soothing cabbage, white potatoes, and sweet potatoes not only were served for dinner, they were the best vegetables for skin care.

Even if you live in a milder climate, remember that winter is the season when normal-to-oily skin needs some tender loving care.

HEALING CABBAGE LEAF CLEANSER

In many European cultures, the women claim that because of cabbage, they have never suffered skin diseases. Rich in sulfur, copper, calcium, and vitamin C, cabbage leaves are soothing, anti-inflammatory, and make a perfect mask.

3 cabbage leaves

½ cup milk

PREPARATION Wrap the cabbage leaves in a paper towel, then microwave on high for 3 minutes. In a blender, mix the leaves and milk together.

APPLICATION Wash your face with this every morning and evening. Rinse off with warm water.

HARVEST CLEANSER

Pumpkins contain antioxidants, which fight the free radicals that are believed to speed up the skin's aging process.

1 slice pumpkin

¼ cup milk

PREPARATION Remove the skin and seeds from the pumpkin slice and cut it into cubes. In a microwave-safe bowl, microwave the pumpkin cubes until they are soft. In a small bowl, mash the pumpkin. In another small bowl, combine 2 tablespoons of the mashed pumpkin with the milk. Add ¼ cup of water and mix well.

APPLICATION Pour a small amount of this onto a clean wet washcloth or sponge. Gently wash your face with this every morning and evening. Rinse with warm water.

ENERGIZE-ME MINT TONER

Mint has a cooling and relaxing effect on the skin. Apple cider vinegar helps maintain an optimal pH balance.

1 cup water

2 mint tea bags

1 teaspoon apple cider vinegar

PREPARATION In a small saucepan, bring the water to a boil. Add the tea bags, then turn off the heat. Steep for 10 minutes, then remove the tea bags. Pour the tea into a clean bowl, and add the vinegar.

APPLICATION Wipe this over your face, using a clean cotton ball, in the evening after cleansing.

NO-PUFFY-EYES POTATO CREAM

In many old-world remedies, the potato was the common ingredient in healing. Curing sunburn and acne, potato juice is also the perfect antidote for puffy, dark under-eye circles.

1 raw potato

1 teaspoon sour cream

1 teaspoon castor oil

PREPARATION In a food processor, liquefy the potato. Blend 1 teaspoon potato juice with the sour cream and oil. Mix well. Refrigerate in a clean container up to 5 days.

APPLICATION Gently apply around the eye area.

LUSCIOUS ORANGE MOISTURIZER

Though it's true that in the summer you don't need to use a moisturizer, for normal-to-oily skin in the winter, it's a must. Otherwise, you will have little dry spots. Greek yogurt is rich and creamy. When tart vitamin C–rich orange juice is added, it's simply luscious!

1 tablespoon orange juice

1 tablespoon Greek yogurt

½ teaspoon cornstarch

PREPARATION In a small bowl, mix together the orange juice, yogurt, and cornstarch until creamy.

APPLICATION Apply a very thin layer of this to your face every morning and evening after cleansing.

HONEY B MOISTURIZER

Sweet, hydrating, and gently exfoliating, honey and baking soda clean without stripping away your skin's natural oils.

1 teaspoon honey

¼ teaspoon baking soda

1 teaspoon vegetable oil

PREPARATION In a small microwave-safe bowl, warm the honey in the microwave for 1 to 2 seconds. Stir in the baking soda, oil, and ¼ cup of water until the ingredients are well mixed.

APPLICATION Apply a very thin layer of this to your face every morning and evening after cleansing. Splash with warm water and pat dry.

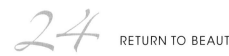

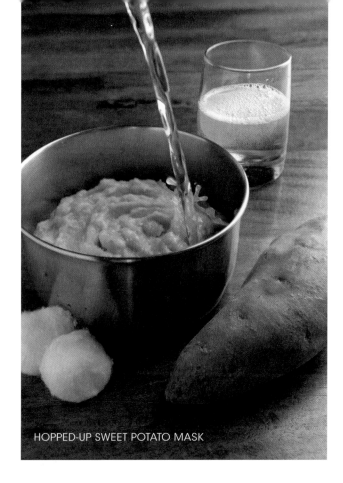

HOPPED-UP SWEET POTATO MASK

HOPPED-UP SWEET POTATO MASK

Sweet potatoes contain vitamin A (beta-carotene) as well as vitamins C and E. These are all effective antioxidants for skin protection. The hops in beer are known to have a relaxing, cleansing effect on the skin.

1 small sweet potato

1 tablespoon beer

PREPARATION Peel and cube the sweet potato and boil it for 10 minutes, drain, then smash it with a fork. In a bowl, combine the potato and the beer. Mix well.

APPLICATION Apply a thick layer of this to your face and neck and relax for 20 minutes. If you'd like, drink the rest of the beer to receive the full effect of the hops! Rinse off with warm water, then apply your moisturizer.

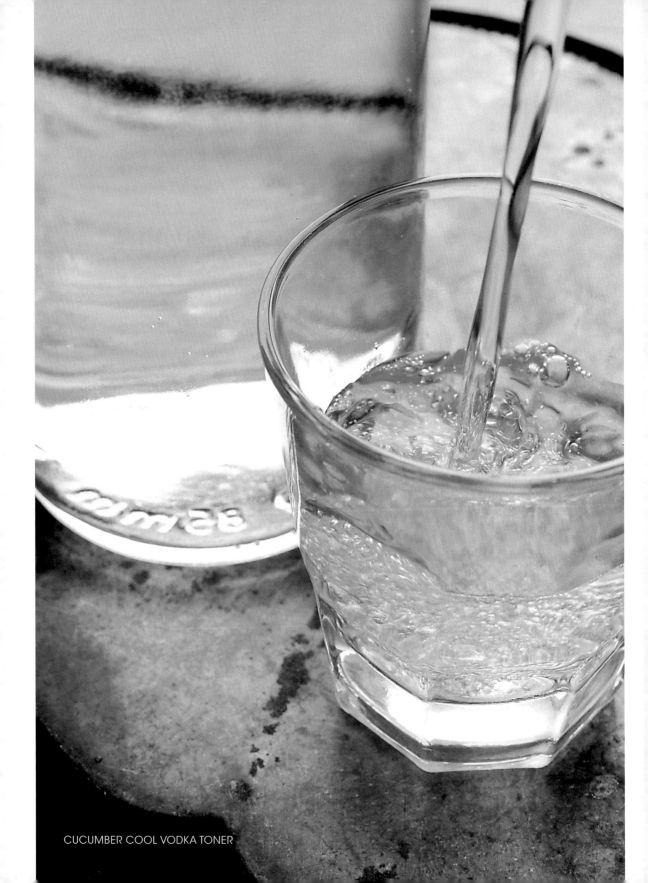

CUCUMBER COOL VODKA TONER

WINTER OILY SKIN

As the earth spins into its darkest season, those of us with oily skin have very little to worry about. We are resilient! Our skin survives the changing elements far better than delicate types.

The following recipes provide the power to keep your skin at its optimum all winter—fresh mint, vodka, and sparkling water.

PRETTY PAPAYA CLEANSER

Papaya is an excellent mild exfoliant—it literally digests dead skin cells. Witch hazel is a gentle astringent.

½ ripe papaya (fresh-frozen if fresh is not available)

5 teaspoons witch hazel

PREPARATION Peel the papaya, cut it in half, and remove the seeds. In a food processor or blender, mix the ingredients together.

APPLICATION Pour a small amount of this onto a clean wet washcloth or sponge. Gently wash your face and neck with this every morning and evening. Rinse with warm water.

JUICY RED CLEANSER

This delicious red juice contains more inflammation-fighting antioxidants than red wine does. Dairy offers soothing exfoliation. Baking soda is alkaline, which neutralizes skin's acidity.

¼ cup pomegranate juice

¼ cup nonfat milk

1 teaspoon baking soda

PREPARATION In a blender, combine the pomegranate juice, milk, and baking soda.

APPLICATION Pour a small amount of this onto a clean wet washcloth or sponge. Gently wash your face and neck with this every morning and evening. Rinse with warm water.

CUCUMBER COOL VODKA TONER

Fresh mint and cucumber supply toning action for the skin. Cucumber is very hydrating.

1 tablespoon chopped fresh mint leaves

¼ cucumber

2 tablespoons vodka

½ cup sparkling mineral water

PREPARATION In a blender, mix together the mint and cucumber. Pour into a clean glass jar and shake well. Add the vodka and mineral water, then strain. Refrigerate up to 1 week.

APPLICATION Gently wipe this over your face, using a clean cotton ball, every morning and evening.

ALMOND OIL EYE CREAM

Almond oil is rich in vitamins and minerals, including vitamins D and E. It's an anti-inflammatory, antiaging skin tonic that softens, nourishes, and soothes the skin.

½ teaspoon almond oil

1 tablespoon plain yogurt

PREPARATION In a small bowl, combine the oil and yogurt. Mix well.

APPLICATION Apply this around the eye area every morning and evening.

HONEY TART MOISTURIZER

Honey hydrates skin without making it shiny. Apple cider vinegar helps maintain your skin's optimal pH balance. Gelatin thickens the recipe.

1 teaspoon honey

2 teaspoons gelatin

½ teaspoon apple cider vinegar

PREPARATION In a small microwave-safe bowl, warm the honey in the microwave. In another small bowl, stir together the gelatin, ½ cup of water, and the vinegar. Add the honey and mix well.

APPLICATION Apply a light coverage of this over your face after cleansing. Splash with warm water and pat dry.

LEMONY FRESH YOGURT MOISTURIZER

In the winter even oily skin needs a little moisture. The lactic acid in the yogurt and the citric acid in the lemon juice will energize your skin. Macadamia nut oil is a light emollient, so you won't feel greasy. This moisturizer is easily absorbed into the skin.

1 tablespoon nonfat plain yogurt

1 teaspoon lemon juice

½ teaspoon cornstarch

1 teaspoon macadamia nut oil

PREPARATION In a small bowl, combine the ingredients and mix well.

APPLICATION Apply a light coverage of this over your face after cleansing.

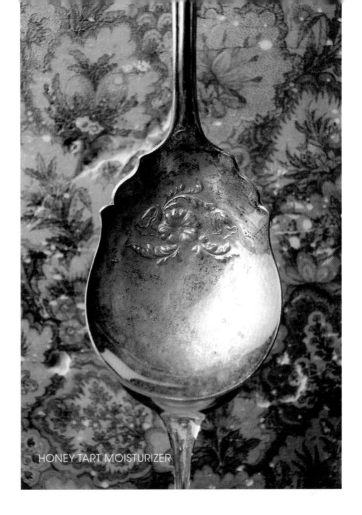

HONEY TART MOISTURIZER

BLUSHING APPLE CARROT MASK

Apples are a happy fruit. With their shot of iron, your skin will glow. Carrots offer protection from the elements. The amino acids in cottage cheese help bleach out uneven skin tone.

1 tablespoon shredded carrot

1 tablespoon shredded apple (unpeeled)

1 tablespoon cottage cheese

PREPARATION In a small bowl, mix together the carrot and apple. Add the cottage cheese and mix well.

APPLICATION Apply a thick layer of this over your face and relax for 20 minutes. Rinse off with warm water, then rinse with cold water. Apply your moisturizer.

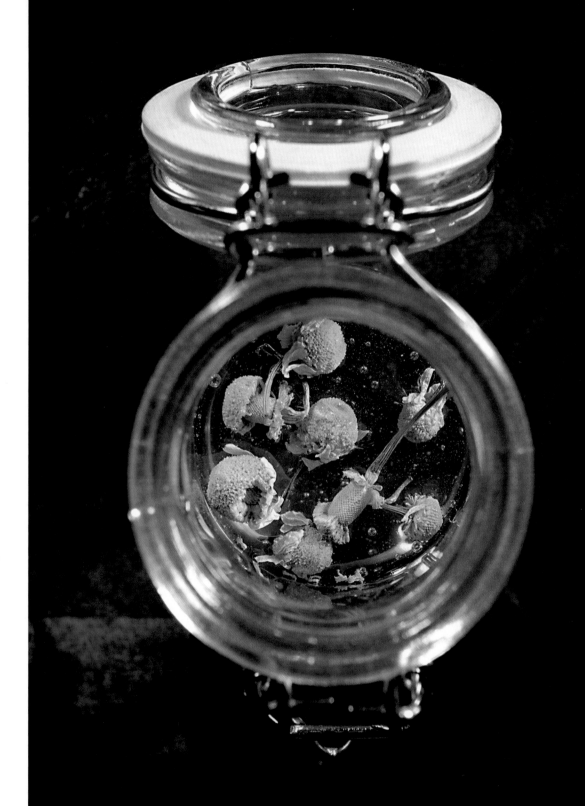

SPRING DRY SKIN

In the spring, flowers need sun and rain to blossom, and you need special attention, too.

Over the years, my more sensitive clients have shared that this is an emotional time for them. For this reason, I've included soothing recipes to calm spring's confused heart as well as its confused dry skin.

Remember to reduce your intake of caffeinated beverages, which can overexcite your system. Try enjoying a cup of chamomile tea while you relax with your mask.

DRY SKIN REGIMEN

SASSY COCONUT PINEAPPLE CLEANSER

In the spring, when your skin needs a little exfoliation, pineapple juice is perfect. It's high in vitamins A, B, and C and folic acid. When the juice is mixed with heavy cream, you have a nice balance. Coconut oil softens, protects, and promotes healing—giving your skin a youthful appearance.

¼ cup heavy cream

1 tablespoon pineapple juice

2 tablespoons coconut oil

PREPARATION In a small bowl, mix the cream with the pineapple juice. Pour in the oil and mix well.

APPLICATION Pour a small amount of this onto a clean wet washcloth or sponge. Gently wash your face with this every morning and evening. Rinse with warm water.

CREAMY WHITE CLEANSER

Egg whites have tonic action, and the lactic acid in sour cream gently exfoliates dead skin cells.

1 egg white

2 tablespoons sour cream

PREPARATION In a small bowl, whisk the egg white until frothy. Add the sour cream and ¼ cup of water and mix well.

APPLICATION Wash your face with this every morning and evening. Rinse off with warm water.

BEAUTIFUL BANANA YOGURT MOISTURIZER

The sweet banana—rich in vitamin A and potassium—is loved by dry skin. Olive oil helps your skin retain moisture all day long.

1 tablespoon plain yogurt

½ banana

1 teaspoon olive oil

PREPARATION In a blender, combine the yogurt, banana, and oil. Mix well.

APPLICATION Apply this to your face every morning and evening after cleansing. Splash with warm water and pat dry.

BUTTERY MANGO MOISTURIZER

Mangoes are high in vitamin C and beta-carotene, and leave skin velvety soft.

1 tablespoon unsalted butter

1 slice mango, peel removed

Pinch of salt

PREPARATION In a small microwave-safe bowl, soften the butter in the microwave for 2 to 3 seconds. In a blender, combine the mango and butter. Add the salt and mix well.

APPLICATION Apply this to your face every morning and evening after cleansing.

AMAZING ALMOND OIL EYE CREAM

Almond oil contains a variety of vitamins and minerals, including vitamins D and E—both good for improving the complexion. It is also an antiaging, anti-irritant, anti-inflammatory skin tonic that is good for all skin types.

1 teaspoon mayonnaise

½ teaspoon almond oil

PREPARATION In a small bowl, combine the mayonnaise and oil. Mix well.

APPLICATION Gently apply a small amount of this around the eye area every morning and evening.

WARM HONEY RISE MASK

Honey is wonderful for older skin. Brewer's yeast is a natural source of B vitamins, which tighten and enhance skin tone. This mask will help you calm down after a long day.

½ tablespoon brewer's yeast

1 teaspoon milk

1 teaspoon honey

PREPARATION In a small bowl, combine the yeast and milk. In a small microwave-safe bowl, warm the honey for 1 or 2 seconds in the microwave, but be careful not to make it too hot. Add the honey to the mixture and mix well.

APPLICATION Cover your face and neck with this, using a cotton ball, and rest until the mask is completely dry. Rinse off with cool water, then apply your moisturizer.

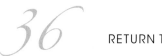

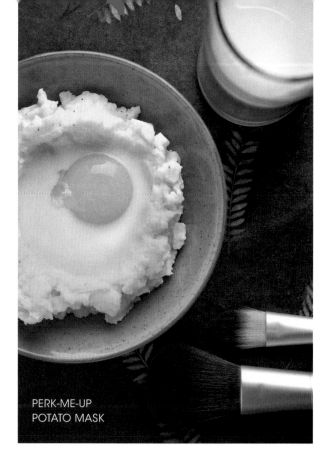

PERK-ME-UP
POTATO MASK

PERK-ME-UP POTATO MASK

Potatoes are the perfect food for waking up a tired face because they contain the mineral copper. Too little copper in your diet can reduce your skin's ability to heal, causing it to become rigid and lifeless. An egg yolk is hydrating. Milk is always soothing.

1 small potato

1 egg yolk

1 tablespoon milk

PREPARATION Preheat the oven to 350°F, then bake the potato for 40 minutes. Peel the skin, then allow it to cool. In a bowl, mash the potato. Add the egg yolk and milk and mix well.

APPLICATION It is better to use this mask while the potato is still warm. Gently apply it to your face and neck and relax for 20 minutes. Rinse off with warm water.

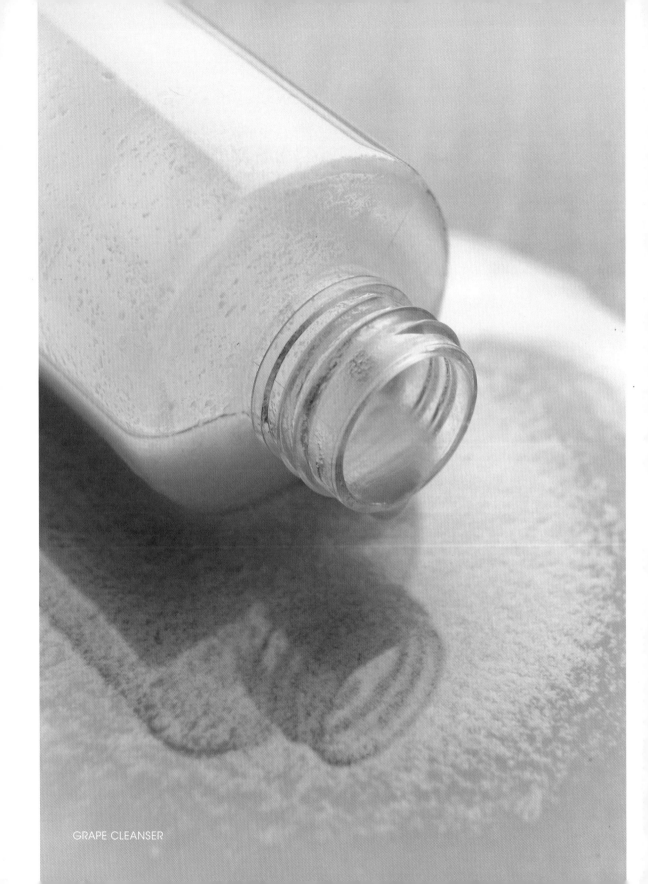

GRAPE CLEANSER

SPRING NORMAL-TO-DRY SKIN

The daylight lasts longer, lifting the somber mood of winter. The lilies on the pond are budding. There's a skip to your step. Is romance in the air?

The following basic recipes offer the magic of spring. A simple routine will keep you shining fresh until summer.

NORMAL-TO-DRY REGIMEN

GRAPE CLEANSER

Grapes are high in minerals and antioxidants. (You can use red or green, whichever are available.) Salt, or baking soda, combined with milk gently exfoliates dead skin cells.

1 cup mashed grapes

1 teaspoon olive oil

½ teaspoon salt (or baking soda)

¼ cup milk

PREPARATION In a blender, combine the grapes, oil, salt (or baking soda), and milk. Mix well.

APPLICATION Gently wash your face with this every morning and evening. Rinse off with warm water.

WARM MILK CLEANSER

Oats contain an antioxidant called phytic acid, which soothes skin. Warm milk is nurturing. This very basic cleanser is all you need to stay clean.

½ cup warm milk

1 tablespoon oatmeal (old-fashioned, not instant or steel-cut)

PREPARATION In a small microwave-safe bowl, warm the milk in the microwave. Stir in the oatmeal and mix well.

APPLICATION Pour a small amount of this onto a clean wet washcloth or sponge. Gently wash your face with this every morning and evening. Rinse with warm water.

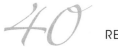

THIRST-QUENCHING TONER

Watermelons are rich in vitamins A, B, and C. This thirst-quenching fruit leaves skin fresh, radiant, and hydrated.

1 cup cubed watermelon

1 tablespoon chopped mint

¼ cup witch hazel

PREPARATION In a blender, combine the watermelon, mint, and witch hazel. Mix well, then strain.

APPLICATION Smooth this over your face, using a clean cotton ball, every evening after cleansing.

TERRIFIC TOMATO MASK

Because normal-to-dry skin doesn't require toner in the spring, this mask contains tomato, which has a natural exfoliating acid that removes the first layer of dead skin. High in vitamin C and the chemical lycopene, this juicy fruit also helps reduce sun damage. Sunflower oil is rich in essential fatty acids. Its light texture is easily absorbed into the skin.

1 ripe tomato

1 teaspoon sunflower oil

1 teaspoon cornstarch

PREPARATION In a blender, puree the tomato. In a small bowl, combine the pureed tomato, oil, and cornstarch to thicken. Mix well.

APPLICATION Cover your face with a thin layer of this mask and relax for 15 minutes. Rinse off with warm water, then apply your moisturizer.

CREAMY MANGO MOISTURIZER

Mangoes are high in vitamin C and antiaging beta-carotene, and leave skin velvety soft.

1 tablespoon mango

1 tablespoon Greek yogurt

1 teaspoon instant oatmeal

PREPARATION In a blender, combine the mango, yogurt, and oatmeal. Mix well.

APPLICATION Cover your face with this in the morning and evening after cleansing. Splash with warm water and pat dry.

HEALING CHAMOMILE MOISTURIZER

Chamomile contains an essential oil known as bisabolol, which has a number of anti-irritant, anti-inflammatory, and antimicrobial properties. This herb comes from the daisy family. It's a healing flower your skin will love! Butter, olive oil, and corn syrup make sure your skin stays supple all day long.

1 tablespoon dried chamomile	1 teaspoon corn syrup
1 teaspoon unsalted butter	½ egg yolk
1 teaspoon olive oil	1 teaspoon vodka

PREPARATION In a small saucepan, add the chamomile to 1 cup of water and bring to a boil. Turn off the heat and steep for 2 hours. In a small bowl, combine the butter, oil, corn syrup, egg yolk, and vodka. Stir well. Strain out the chamomile leaves and add the extract to the mixture. Mix well.

APPLICATION Cover your face with this in the morning and evening after cleansing. Splash with warm water and pat dry.

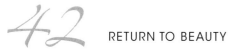

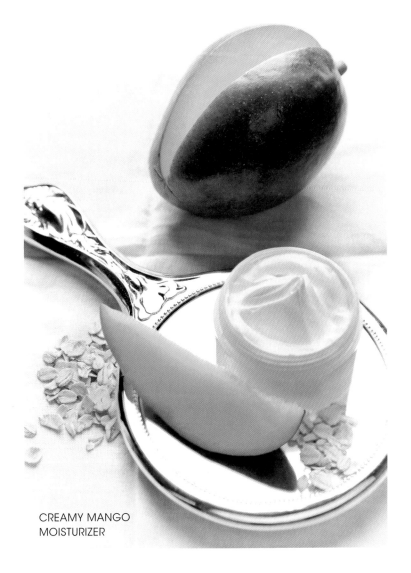

CREAMY MANGO
MOISTURIZER

EXCELLENT VITAMIN E EYE CREAM

Vitamin E's rich oil is a complete moisturizer for the area around your eyes.

2 vitamin E oil capsules

PREPARATION Cut off the tips of the capsules and squeeze the oil onto the tip of your finger.

APPLICATION Massage this gently around the eye area.

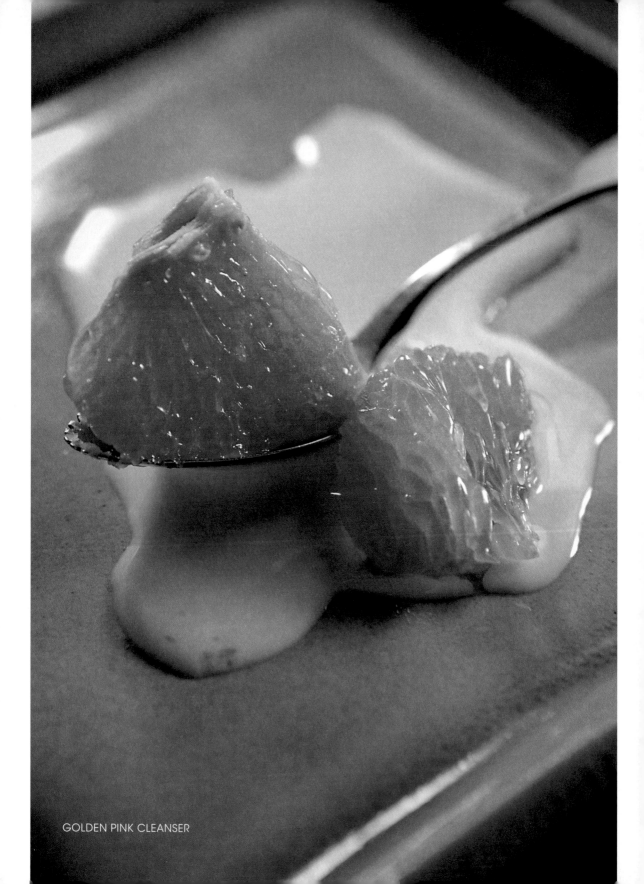

GOLDEN PINK CLEANSER

SPRING NORMAL-TO-OILY SKIN

With the onset of warmer weather, normal-to-oily skin will stay beautiful only if it's kept clean.

The following recipes reflect the need for more aggressive ingredients in order to keep breakouts at bay. Salt and orange peel may sound like harsh components, but my grandmother used them on me when I was a young girl and I loved them. They made my face tingle.

After years of experimenting with these ingredients, I have learned their true benefits. These recipes don't only make your face tingle, they tighten your skin!

NORMAL-TO-OILY SKIN REGIMEN

FROTHY MILK CLEANSER

Milk is an instant skin beautifier—inside and out. Carbonated water activates the salt, assuring thorough, gentle cleansing.

¼ cup milk

¼ cup carbonated water

1 teaspoon salt

PREPARATION In a clean plastic bottle, combine the ingredients. Shake well to mix.

APPLICATION Pour a small amount of this onto a clean wet washcloth or sponge. Gently wash your face with this every morning and evening. Rinse with warm water.

GOLDEN PINK CLEANSER

Grapefruits contain citric acid, which rejuvenates skin and closes pores. They also contain fructose and vitamins A, C, and D. The juice assists in collagen production, which supports healthier, smoother skin.

2 tablespoons grapefruit juice

½ teaspoon baking soda

2 tablespoons nonfat plain yogurt

PREPARATION In a small bowl, combine the grapefruit juice, baking soda, and yogurt. Blend well.

APPLICATION Pour a small amount of this onto a clean wet washcloth or sponge. Gently wash your face with this every morning and evening. Rinse with warm water.

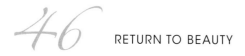

ORANGE YOU GORGEOUS VODKA TONER

Orange peel is a rich source of flavonoids, which are potent antioxidants. Vodka's gentle, natural alcohol closes pores.

1 tablespoon grated orange zest

2 tablespoons vodka

PREPARATION In a clean plastic container, mix the zest, vodka, and ¼ cup of water. Shake well, then strain.

APPLICATION Gently wipe this over your face using a clean cotton ball.

SO DELICIOUS! COCOA BUTTER EYE CREAM

Vitamin E is easily absorbed by the skin, and it reduces the appearance of fine lines and wrinkles. Its antioxidant activity fights free radicals.

½ tablespoon cocoa butter

2 vitamin E capsules

PREPARATION In a small microwave-safe bowl, liquefy the cocoa butter by heating it for several seconds in the microwave or in a water bath. Cut off the tips of the capsules. In a small bowl, combine the butter and oil. Test for temperature.

APPLICATION Gently apply a thin layer of this around the eye area.

LEMON FIGGY MOISTURIZER

Lemon is a great source of citric acid, which closes pores. Figs contain natural humectants—the perfect skin hydrator.

1 tablespoon chopped black figs

1 tablespoon low-fat sour cream

1 tablespoon lemon juice

PREPARATION In a blender, combine the figs and the sour cream and mix well. Add the lemon juice and blend again until creamy.

APPLICATION Apply a thin layer of this over your face in the morning and evening after cleansing.

SWEET LILY MILK MOISTURIZER

Lilies smell terrific while they smooth your skin.

½ cup chopped lily flowers

½ cup milk

½ teaspoon honey

1 teaspoon sunflower oil

PREPARATION In a small saucepan, cook the lily in the milk over low heat for 5 minutes, then strain. In a blender, combine the lily milk, honey, and oil. Mix until creamy.

APPLICATION Cover your face with this in the morning and evening after cleansing. Splash with warm water and pat dry.

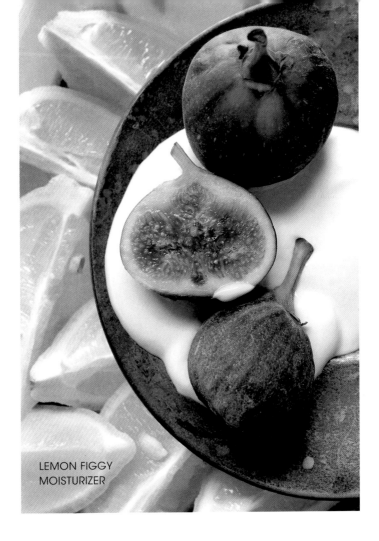

LEMON FIGGY
MOISTURIZER

GORGEOUS GIRL GREEN PEA MASK

Green peas are good for blood circulation. They contain vitamins A and C. Mix them with plain yogurt, and your skin will love this colorful mask!

2 tablespoons frozen green peas

1 tablespoon plain yogurt

PREPARATION Bring the peas to a boil in ½ cup of water. Cook for 5 minutes, drain, and allow to cool. In a blender, combine the peas and yogurt. Mix well.

APPLICATION While this is still warm, apply a thick layer to your face and neck and relax for 20 minutes. Rinse off with warm water, then apply your moisturizer.

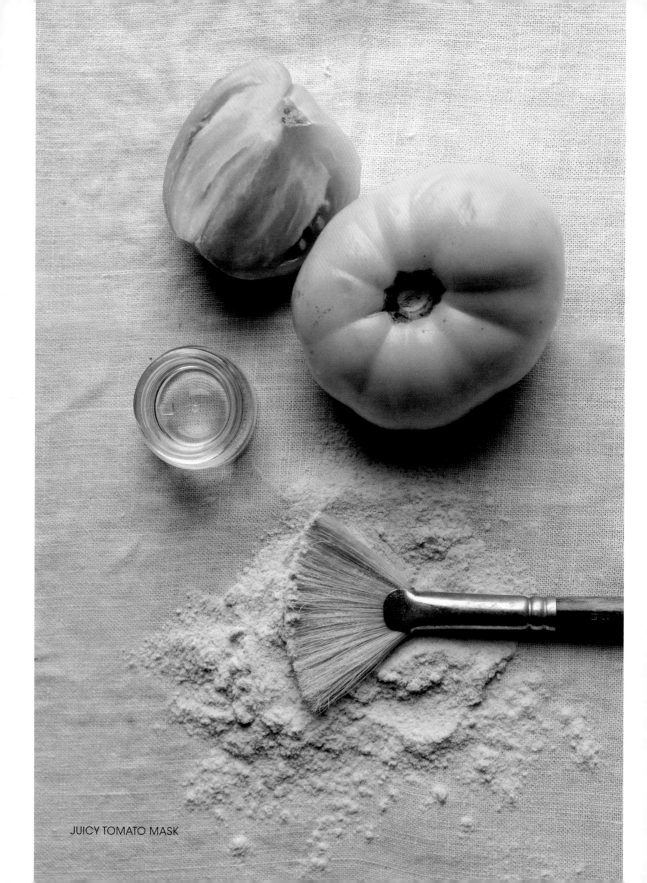

JUICY TOMATO MASK

SPRING OILY SKIN

Quick—here comes the sun! The long-awaited sunshine breaking through the clouds can also be the beginning of an oily skin breakout.

Now is the time to quickly step up your routine with dedication—and high-powered ingredients like apple cider vinegar, cucumbers, and tomatoes.

OILY SKIN REGIMEN

MILK AND BAKING SODA BASIC CLEANSER

This all-natural cleanser is rich in protein and lactic acid—a great detoxifier. Baking soda is alkaline, neutralizing acidity. When mixed with water, it's the perfect way to keep oily skin sparkling clean all spring.

1 tablespoon baking soda

¼ cup milk

PREPARATION In a small bowl, mix the baking soda into the milk. Add 2 tablespoons of water and mix well.

APPLICATION Pour a small amount of this onto a clean wet washcloth or sponge. Gently wash your face and neck with this every morning and evening. Rinse off with warm water.

SALTY WHITE CLEANSER

Egg white offers tonic action. Sea salt is great for oily skin and won't cause irritation—it will only leave it glowing.

1 egg white

2 tablespoons plain yogurt

½ teaspoon sea salt

PREPARATION In a small bowl, whisk the egg white until frothy. In a separate bowl, combine the yogurt and salt, then fold in the egg white.

APPLICATION Wash your face and neck with this every morning and evening. Rinse off with warm water.

CUCUMBER RESTORATION TONER

Oily skin always needs a toner. Cucumber acts as the perfect astringent when combined with witch hazel and apple cider vinegar. It's a wonderful skin refresher—restoring acidity and fighting off blackheads.

½ cucumber

¼ cup witch hazel

1 tablespoon apple cider vinegar

PREPARATION Peel the cucumber and then shred it. In a clean glass jar, combine the shredded cucumber, witch hazel, and vinegar. Shake well to mix, then strain into a clean container. Refrigerate for up to 1 week.

APPLICATION Wipe your face with this gently, using a clean cotton ball, every morning and evening.

JUICY TOMATO MASK

Because of its highly acidic properties, the tomato is a great fruit for oily skin. It's also high in vitamins A, B, and C. Egg yolks contain lecithin and are a natural emollient. Cornstarch binds the ingredients.

1 ripe tomato

1 egg yolk

1 teaspoon cornstarch

PREPARATION In a blender, combine the tomato and egg yolk and mix well. Pour the mixture into a bowl, then slowly add the cornstarch to thicken.

APPLICATION Apply this to your face and neck and relax for 20 minutes. Rinse off with warm water, then apply your moisturizer.

MAGIC MELON MOISTURIZER

Melons are cooling and hydrating. They contain vitamins A, B, and C and natural sugars, which are healing for the skin. Lemon is good for skin tone. This moisturizer balances skin's pH.

1 slice honeydew melon

1 teaspoon sunflower oil

1 teaspoon lemon juice

PREPARATION Peel the melon, then puree it in a food processor or blender. Add the oil and lemon juice and blend until creamy.

APPLICATION Apply a very thin layer of this over your face and neck every morning and evening after cleansing.

TANGO MANGO MOISTURIZER

Mangoes are high in vitamin C and antiaging beta-carotene.

½ mango

1 tablespoon nonfat sour cream

1 teaspoon apple cider vinegar

PREPARATION Remove the seed and skin from the mango. In a blender, combine the mango, sour cream, and vinegar. Blend until creamy.

APPLICATION Apply a very thin layer of this over your face and neck every morning and evening after cleansing.

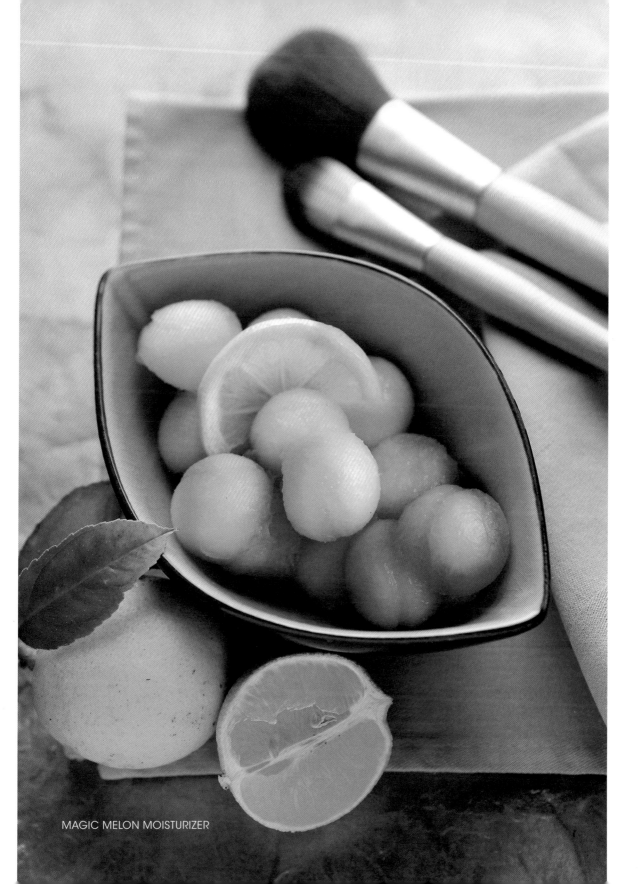

MAGIC MELON MOISTURIZER

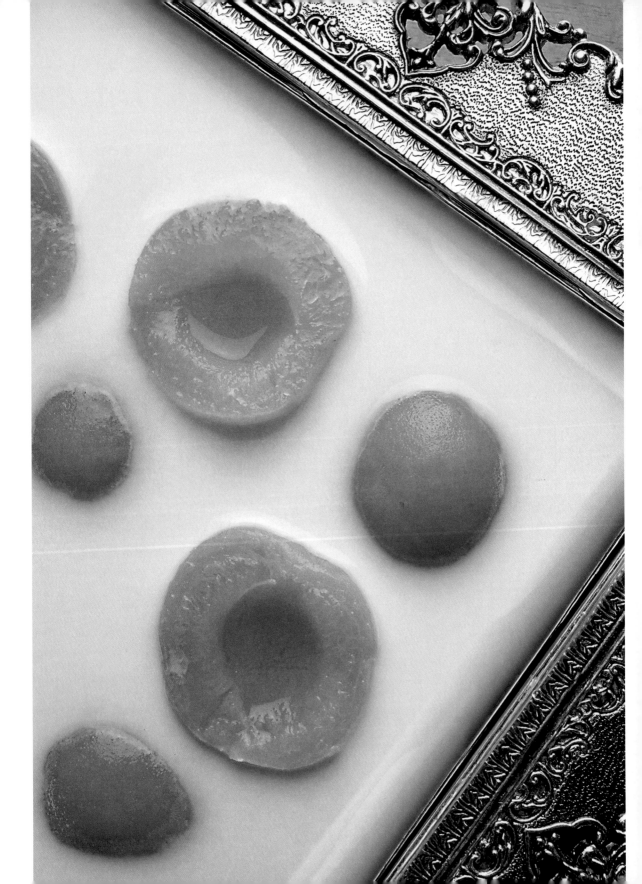

SUMMER DRY SKIN

Blue sky, fresh air, and plenty of sunshine—ah, the joyful benefits of summer!

During the hot months, I like to introduce slightly more aggressive exfoliants for dry skin. Sugar, fresh apricots, lemons, and carrot juice are all high in citric acids that safely slough away dead skin cells. They also help prevent wrinkles, and calm and tone your skin.

Remember to scrub once or twice a month to receive the full benefits of your moisturizer.

DRY SKIN REGIMEN

LEMON 'N' HONEY CLEANSER

Milk is the best cleanser for skin. Honey naturally exfoliates. The vitamin C in lemon juice helps produce a rosy complexion.

¼ cup milk

1 tablespoon honey

1 teaspoon lemon juice

PREPARATION In a small bowl, combine the milk and honey and mix well. Add the lemon juice and mix well.

APPLICATION Pour a small amount of this onto a clean wet washcloth or sponge. Gently wash your face with this every morning and evening. Rinse with warm water.

ROSE RED CLEANSER

Roses and apples smooth your skin and bring a healthy color to your cheeks.

½ cup rose petals

½ cup apple juice

1 teaspoon honey

PREPARATION In a small saucepan, bring the petals and apple juice to a boil. Steep for 10 minutes. Strain, then mix with honey.

APPLICATION Pour a small amount of this onto a clean wet washcloth or sponge. Gently wash your face with this every morning and evening. Rinse with warm water.

CALM CHAMOMILE TONER

Chamomile not only eases anxiety, it has anti-inflammatory and antimicrobial properties. This flower can also be used for combating deeper skin issues, like psoriasis and eczema. Vodka is a gentle antiseptic.

1 chamomile tea bag

½ teaspoon vodka

PREPARATION In a small saucepan, slowly boil the tea bag in 2 cups of water for 10 minutes. Remove the tea bag, allow the tea to cool, then add the vodka.

APPLICATION After cleansing at night, wipe this on your face gently, using a clean cotton ball.

BUBBLY RASILICIOUS MASK

Luscious raspberries exude powers of renewal. Rich in vitamins C and A as well as manganese, this fruit offers a calming and toning effect.

15 raspberries

3 tablespoons milk

1 teaspoon olive oil

1 teaspoon sparkling mineral water

PREPARATION In a small bowl, mash the raspberries. Add the milk and then the olive oil. Mix well, then add the sparkling water and mix well again.

APPLICATION Apply a thin layer of this to your face and relax for 20 minutes. Rinse off with warm water, then apply your moisturizer.

CARROT NUTTY SMOOTH MOISTURIZER

Nature's defender, carrots help balance the pH of your skin's surface. When combined with coconut and yogurt, they make a mask that rejuvenates aging skin.

1 tablespoon nonfat plain yogurt

1 tablespoon carrot juice

½ teaspoon coconut oil

PREPARATION In a small bowl, combine the yogurt and carrot juice and mix well. Add the coconut oil and mix well again.

APPLICATION Gently cover your face with this every morning and evening after cleansing.

COOL 'N' RICH MOISTURIZER

Cucumbers are hydrating and cause toning action in skin.

1 small cucumber

1 tablespoon nonfat plain yogurt

½ teaspoon cornstarch

PREPARATION In a blender, puree the cucumber. In a small bowl, combine 1 tablespoon of the cucumber and the yogurt. Stir in the cornstarch and mix well.

APPLICATION Gently cover your face with this every morning and evening after cleansing.

COOL GREEN EYE CREAM

Avocados are abundant in essential oils and B-complex vitamins that nourish skin inside and out. Niacin (vitamin B$_3$) is especially important for healthy skin.

1 small cucumber

½ teaspoon mashed avocado

PREPARATION In a blender, puree the cucumber. In a bowl, mix 1 teaspoon of the pureed cucumber and the avocado.

APPLICATION Apply this gently to the eye area every morning and evening.

SWEETIE SUGAR SCRUB

Sugar gently sloughs away dead skin. Egg whites have tonic action. Use this twice a month.

1 egg white

1 teaspoon sugar

½ teaspoon cottage cheese

PREPARATION In a small bowl, beat the egg white. Add the sugar and cottage cheese and mix well.

APPLICATION Using your fingers, gently rub this into your T-zone (nose, chin, and forehead). Rinse off with warm water.

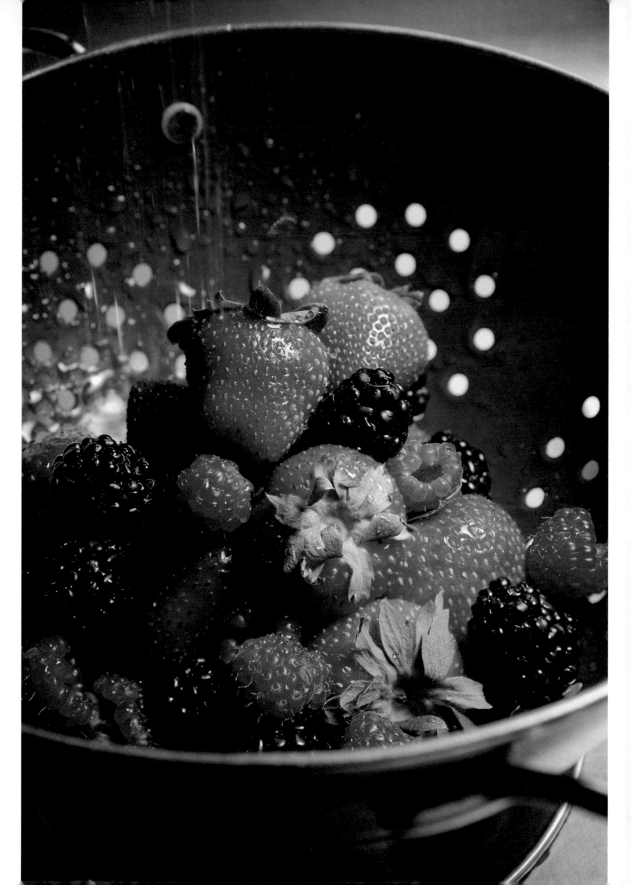

SUMMER NORMAL-TO-DRY SKIN

Picnics on the beach, barbecues, and hiking through the park—summer has finally arrived!

Normal-to-oily skin enjoys summer's treats—strawberries, pineapples, and avocado. Any citrus combination will perk you up right away.

Remember to cleanse and moisturize to keep your skin from developing dry spots.

NORMAL-TO-DRY SKIN REGIMEN

CABBAGE MILK CLEANSER

Rich in sulfur, calcium, and vitamin C, cabbage is excellent for tending to skin's needs. Dairy naturally exfoliates dead skin cells.

2 large cabbage leaves

¼ cup milk

1 teaspoon olive oil

PREPARATION Wrap the leaves in a paper towel and microwave for 3 minutes. In a blender, combine the leaves, milk, and oil. Blend to a thick consistency.

APPLICATION Wash your face with this every morning and evening. Rinse off with warm water.

CHAMOMILE CLEANSER

Chamomile has anti-irritant, anti-inflammatory, and antimicrobial properties.

1 teaspoon dried chamomile

1 teaspoon oatmeal (old-fashioned, not instant or steel-cut)

PREPARATION In a small saucepan, bring the dried chamomile and ½ cup of water to a boil. Steep for 10 minutes, then strain. In a blender, mix the liquid and oatmeal until creamy.

APPLICATION Pour a small amount of this onto a clean wet washcloth or sponge. Gently wash your face with this every morning and evening. Rinse with warm water.

PERFECT PINEAPPLE TONER

In the summer, you need to use a toner. The enzymes in pineapple make this the perfect refresher—without stripping skin's natural oils. Vitamin C is added to boost the anti-inflammatory, antiseptic quality.

1 vitamin C tablet

1 teaspoon pineapple juice

PREPARATION In a small saucepan, bring 1 cup of water to a boil. Add the vitamin C tablet and allow it to dissolve. Let it cool, then pour it into a clean plastic bottle. Add the pineapple juice and shake well.

APPLICATION Gently wipe this over your face as needed using a clean cotton ball.

A+ AVOCADO EYE CREAM

Rich in essential oils and nourishing B-complex vitamins including niacin (vitamin B_3), avocado offers the same benefits as top-of-the line cosmetics.

1 teaspoon avocado (scooped out from a halved avocado)

¼ teaspoon plain yogurt

PREPARATION In a small bowl, mix the avocado and yogurt. *Tip:* Wrap the avocado with the pit in a plastic bag and refrigerate for use all week.

APPLICATION Massage this gently around the eye area.

TARTY RED BERRY MOISTURIZER

The tiny little cranberry packs a punch of vitamins that protect skin from bacteria in the summer months. Mildly acidic, the berry also offers gentle exfoliation. When egg yolk and butter are combined, skin stays hydrated.

2 tablespoons cranberries

½ egg yolk

1 teaspoon unsalted butter

PREPARATION In a small saucepan, boil the cranberries for 3 to 4 minutes to soften them, allow them to cool, then mash them with a fork in a small bowl. In a small microwave-safe bowl, soften the butter in the microwave for 1 to 2 seconds. Add the egg yolk and butter to the mashed cranberries and beat well.

APPLICATION Cover your face with a thin layer of this every morning and evening after cleansing. Splash with warm water and pat dry.

PAPAYA NUT MOISTURIZER

Papaya enzymes literally digest dead skin cells as well as reduce age spots and fine lines. Almond oil is an anti-inflammatory, antiaging skin tonic that softens, nourishes, and soothes skin.

½ papaya

1 teaspoon almond oil

1 tablespoon plain yogurt

PREPARATION Remove the skin and seeds from the papaya. In a blender, combine the papaya, oil, and yogurt. Mix until creamy.

APPLICATION Cover your face with a thin layer of this every morning and evening after cleansing.

POSITIVELY STRAWBERRY MASK

Strawberries are packed with vitamin C. They also contain salicylic acid, which removes dead skin cells. Buttermilk has natural gentle alpha hydroxy acid. After a long day, even the scent of this mask rejuvenates.

2 tablespoons mashed strawberries

1 teaspoon honey

1 tablespoon buttermilk

PREPARATION In a small bowl, blend the strawberries, honey, and buttermilk until creamy.

APPLICATION Cover your face and neck with a thin layer of this and relax for 15 minutes. Rinse off with warm water, then apply your moisturizer.

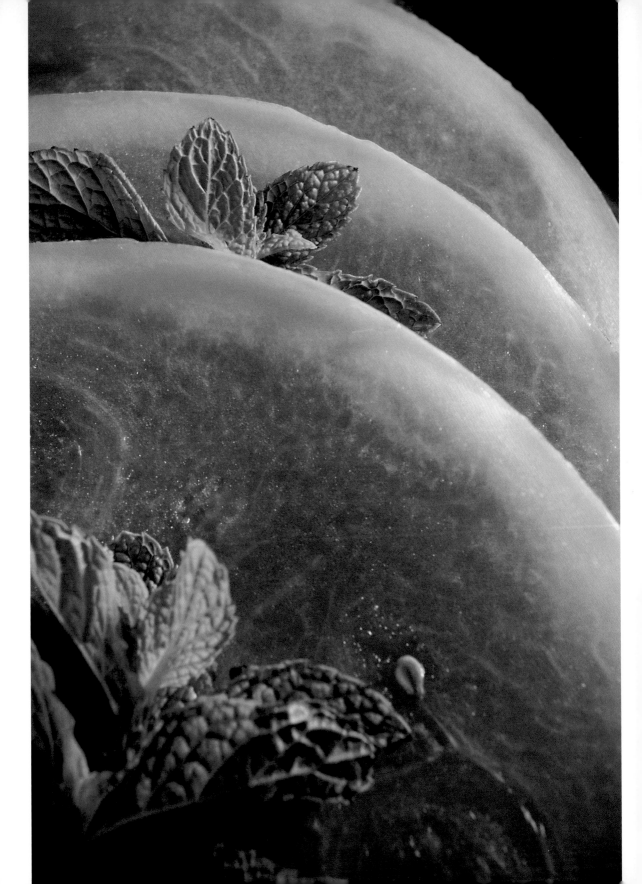

SUMMER NORMAL-TO-OILY SKIN

This is the season filled with fruits that renew us inside and out—like papayas and watermelon. Bursting with life, these natural fruit acids act as mild exfoliants—bringing a natural freshness to your life.

Plus, the sweet scent of coconut oil puts you in that happy summer mood!

NORMAL-TO-OILY SKIN REGIMEN

SALTY SPARKLING ORANGE CLEANSER

Oranges are packed with antiaging vitamin C. Mineral water and sea salt cleanse away impurities without harming your skin.

½ orange, skin intact

¼ cup mineral water

1 teaspoon sea salt

PREPARATION In a blender, combine the orange, water, and salt. Mix well.

APPLICATION Pour a small amount of this onto a clean wet washcloth or sponge. Gently wash your face with this every morning and evening. Rinse with cold water.

CARROT JUICY JUICE CLEANSER

Carrot juice is great for your face in the hot sun—the beta-carotene lessens your chances of getting sunburned. Baking soda is a gentle cleanser, and when it's mixed with the lactic acid in milk, blemishes are kept at bay.

¼ cup nonfat milk

1 teaspoon baking soda

2 tablespoons carrot juice

PREPARATION In a clean glass bottle, combine the ingredients. Shake well to mix.

APPLICATION Pour a small amount of this onto a clean wet washcloth or sponge. Gently wash your face with this every morning and evening. Rinse with cold water.

WICKEDLY WONDERFUL WATERMELON TONER

Watermelons are rich in vitamins A, B, and C. The antiseptic quality of witch hazel is a daily must-do for normal-to-oily skin in the summer. Vodka enhances the drying effect without drying out skin.

2 tablespoons witch hazel

2 tablespoons vodka

¼ cup watermelon juice

PREPARATION Combine the ingredients in a clean plastic (or glass) bottle. Shake well.

APPLICATION Wipe your face with a clean cotton ball dipped in this several times a day as needed.

I LIKE DA COCONUT OIL EYE CREAM

Coconut oil helps skin retain its moisture. Vitamin E protects skin.

2 vitamin E capsules

1 tablespoon coconut oil

PREPARATION Cut off the tips of the capsules. In a small bowl, combine the oils.

APPLICATION Massage this gently around the eye area only in the morning.

HONEY, IT'S DELICIOUS WALNUT SCRUB

Honey has natural properties that alleviate redness and calm irritated skin. Walnuts are packed with beta-carotene and vitamin E, as well as a healthy dose of alpha-linolenic acid, which helps skin stay soft, smooth, and supple. Tip: Lick your fingers when you've finished— this scrub is delicious!

1 tablespoon ground walnuts

½ tablespoon plain yogurt

1 tablespoon honey

PREPARATION In a small bowl, combine the ground walnuts and yogurt and mix well. Add the honey and mix well again.

APPLICATION Massage this gently over your face, paying special attention to the T-zone (chin, nose, and forehead). Try using the scrub in the shower, when pores are more open. After massaging it into your skin, leave it on for another 5 minutes while you shave your legs. Rinse off with warm water.

LOVELY LEMON EGG-WHITE MASK

Like dairy, oatmeal provides gentle, skin-renewing exfoliation. Egg whites tighten pores. Lemons refresh and are a natural exfoliant.

1 egg white

1 tablespoon oatmeal (old-fashioned, not instant or steel-cut)

1 tablespoon lemon juice

PREPARATION In a small bowl, whisk the egg white until frothy. Add the oatmeal and lemon juice and mix well.

APPLICATION Apply a thin layer of this over your face and neck and relax for 20 minutes. Rinse off with warm water, then rinse with cold water. Apply your moisturizer.

NUTRITIOUS NECTARINE MOISTURIZER

The juicy nectarine is a great source of vitamin A and vitamin C—pure nutrition for your skin. Almond oil aids in skin softening.

1 nectarine

1 tablespoon nonfat plain yogurt

1 teaspoon almond oil

PREPARATION Peel and core the nectarine. Boil in 1 cup of water for 5 to 7 minutes, drain, and allow to cool. In a blender, combine the nectarine, yogurt, and oil. Blend until creamy.

APPLICATION Cover your face with a thin layer of this after cleansing.

CREAMY PEACH MOISTURIZER

Peaches improve the complexion. Peach skin offers astringent action, which tightens pores. Milk is soothing and hydrating and gently exfoliates.

¼ peach

1 tablespoon milk

¼ teaspoon flour

PREPARATION Cube the peach. In a blender, combine the peach and milk. Pour into a bowl, and add the flour to thicken.

APPLICATION Cover your face with a thin layer of this after cleansing.

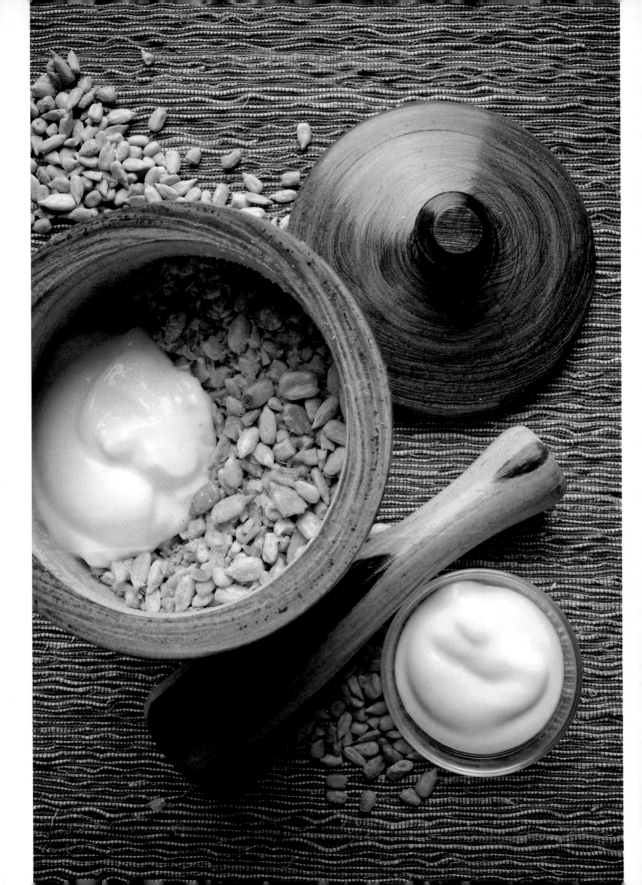

SUMMER OILY SKIN

Oh, how the lazy days of summer can wreak havoc on the beautiful skin you worked so hard the rest of the year to maintain! If you're a member of the oily skin club, you have specific challenges during hot and humid weather.

In the Old Country, people used sand and pickles to make acne treatments for the summer months. Never fear, my grandmother's recipes are much more appealing—they call for grapefruit, vodka with rose petals, grapes, and sunflower seeds.

These recipes keep blackheads at bay—and make your regimen comfortable and easy.

Please note: No moisturizer for oily skin in the summer.

OILY SKIN REGIMEN

GRAPEFRUIT REFRESH CLEANSER

Grapefruits contain citric acid, which rejuvenates skin and closes pores. They also contain fructose and vitamins A, C, and D.

¼ cup grapefruit juice

1 tablespoon olive oil

½ teaspoon flour

PREPARATION In a blender, combine the grapefruit juice and oil. Mix well. Pour into a bowl, and add the flour to thicken.

APPLICATION Pour a small amount of this onto a clean wet washcloth or sponge. Gently wash your face with this every morning and evening. Rinse with warm water.

BUBBLY STRAWBERRY CLEANSER

Strawberries are packed with vitamin C. They also contain salicylic acid, which removes dead skin cells.

3 large strawberries

½ cup mineral water

¼ teaspoon baking soda

PREPARATION In a blender, combine the strawberries, water, and baking soda. Mix well.

APPLICATION Pour a small amount of this onto a clean wet washcloth or sponge. Gently wash your face with this every morning and evening. Rinse with warm water.

BLUSHING ROSE VODKA TONER

Lemon has citric acid in it, and the vodka is ethanol. Together, they create a strong anti-bacterial combination. The rose petals calm and soften skin, adding a blush to your cheeks.

3 tablespoons chopped rose petals

½ cup vodka

2 tablespoons lemon juice

PREPARATION In a clean glass container, combine the petals, vodka, and lemon juice. Set aside for 24 hours, then refrigerate for up to 1 week. Shake well, then strain.

APPLICATION Wipe this over your face as needed, using a clean cotton ball. Remember: Use toner after exercising.

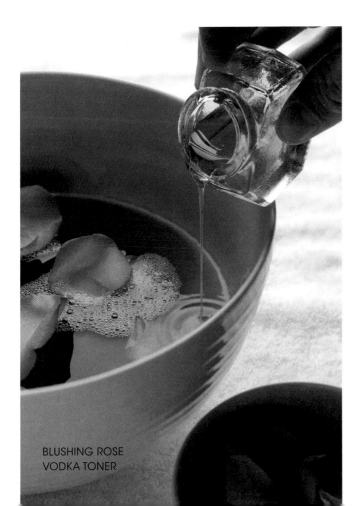

BLUSHING ROSE
VODKA TONER

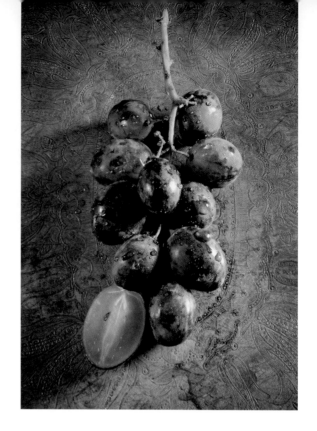

CLEOPATRA'S BLACK GRAPE SCRUB

Black grapes are high in minerals and antioxidants. Sunflower seeds are an excellent source of vitamin E.

1 tablespoon raw sunflower seeds

5 black grapes

½ teaspoon baking soda

1 teaspoon distilled water

PREPARATION Grind the seeds to a powder. In a food processor or blender, combine the sunflower seed powder, grapes, and baking soda. Pour in the distilled water and mix well.

APPLICATION Once or twice a week, massage this over your face, paying attention to the T-zone (nose, chin, and forehead area). If your skin is especially oily, leave the scrub on for 5 minutes in the shower while you shave your legs. Rinse off with warm water, then rinse with cold water.

PINEAPPLE SCRUMPTIOUS MASK

Egg whites make this a great pore-refining mask. Pineapples remove dead skin cells and polish the skin's surface.

1 slice of pineapple, rind removed

1 egg white

1 tablespoon honey

½ teaspoon oatmeal (old-fashioned, not instant or steel-cut)

PREPARATION In a blender or food processor, puree the pineapple. In a small bowl, whisk the egg white until frothy. Add the pureed pineapple, honey, and oatmeal to the egg white and mix well.

APPLICATION Cover your face and neck with this and relax for 20 minutes. Rinse off with warm water.

CARROTS 'N' CRÈME EYE CREAM

Carrots are a good source of beta-carotene—very rejuvenating! Sour cream and cottage cheese lighten dark under-eye circles.

½ teaspoon sour cream

½ tablespoon cottage cheese

½ teaspoon carrot juice

PREPARATION In a small bowl, combine the sour cream and cottage cheese. Add the carrot juice and mix well.

APPLICATION Gently apply a small amount of this around the entire eye area in the evening after cleansing.

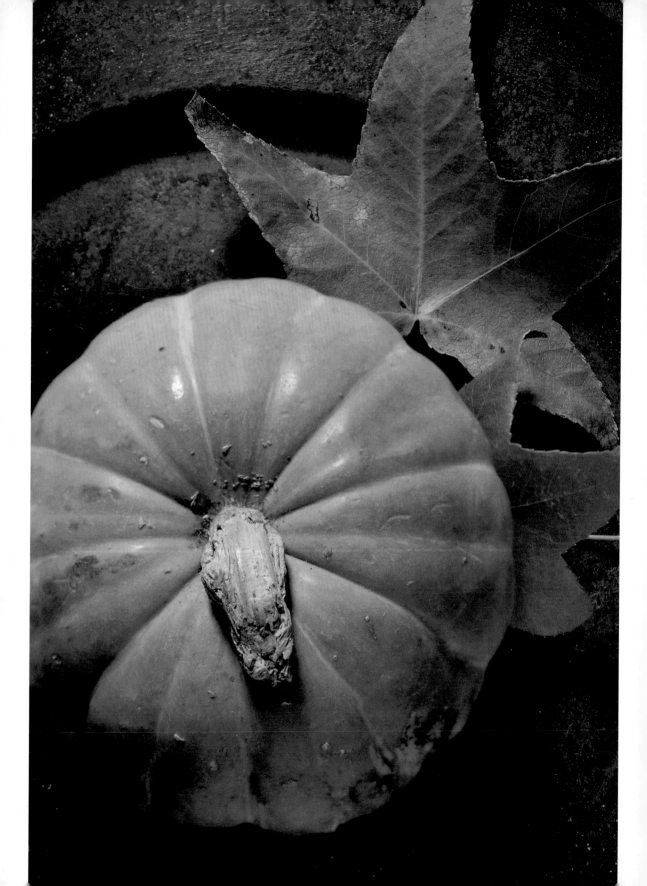

FALL DRY SKIN

There's a chill in the air!

Fall is my favorite season. The yummy scent of pumpkins or fresh cranberries simmering on the stove fills the house. These two great fruits are not only a treat for the senses, they are the perfect foods to moisturize and protect dry skin during bitter-cold or dry weather.

Plus, they'll keep you looking rosy and delicious!

DRY SKIN REGIMEN

HONEY, I GOT THE MILK CLEANSER

Oatmeal is a great cleanser for dry skin. Milk and honey offer gentle exfoliation and give this recipe a creamy texture.

1 tablespoon oatmeal (old-fashioned, not instant or steel-cut)

¼ cup milk

1 tablespoon honey

PREPARATION In a food processor or blender, combine the oatmeal, milk, and honey. Mix until smooth.

APPLICATION Gently wash your face in the evening with a small amount of this. Rinse off with warm water.

SIMMERING PUMPKIN CLEANSER

Pumpkins are high in the mineral zinc, which is a mild astringent that tightens body tissue. It also has anti-inflammatory properties.

1 pumpkin wedge (to make 1 cup shredded)

1 teaspoon salt

PREPARATION Peel and shred the pumpkin. In a small saucepan, bring 1 cup of water, the pumpkin, and salt to a boil. Reduce the heat and simmer until the pumpkin is soft. Drain. In a blender, puree the cooked pumpkin until creamy. Allow to cool.

APPLICATION Gently wash your face in the evening with a small amount of this. Rinse off with warm water.

CRANBERRIES 'N' APPLES MASK

The beautiful dark red cranberry contains an antioxidant that helps reduce the risk of skin cancer. Because of its mild acidic quality, this fruit also offers gentle skin exfoliation.

5 tablespoons fresh cranberries

1 apple, unpeeled

1 tablespoon flaxseed oil

PREPARATION In a small saucepan, boil the cranberries for 5 minutes in 1 cup of water. Mash them and then allow them to cool. Shred the apple. Mix the fruits together, then add the flaxseed oil to bind.

APPLICATION Apply a thick layer and relax for 20 minutes. Rinse off with warm water, then apply your moisturizer.

PUMPKIN HAPPY FACE MASK

Jack-o'-lanterns aren't just for Halloween. Pumpkins make a great face food for dry skin in the fall. High in the mineral zinc, as well as in beta-carotene and vitamin C, pumpkin contains antioxidants that fight the free radicals believed to speed up skin's aging process.

1 pumpkin wedge

1 tablespoon olive oil

PREPARATION Remove the rind and chop the pumpkin into 10 cubes. Boil the pumpkin cubes in water for 10 minutes, drain, then mash them and allow to cool. Combine 2 tablespoons of mashed pumpkin with the oil and mix well.

APPLICATION Gently apply this to your face and neck and relax for 20 minutes. Rinse off with warm water, then apply your moisturizer.

TANGERINE DREAM MOISTURIZER

Tangerines are rich in vitamin C and offer strong antioxidants. This moisturizer refreshes and reenergizes skin.

¼ tangerine, peel and pith removed

1 tablespoon sour cream

½ teaspoon flour

1 teaspoon rose oil

PREPARATION In a blender, combine the tangerine, sour cream, flour, and oil. Mix well.

APPLICATION Apply this to your face every morning and evening after cleansing.

CARROT PROTECTOR MOISTURIZER

Your skin loves carrots year-round. High in vitamins and minerals, this vegetable prevents dryness. Gentle yogurt and olive oil combine to create the perfect emollient for hydration.

½ carrot, unpeeled and chopped

1 teaspoon plain yogurt

½ teaspoon olive oil

PREPARATION Boil the carrot in 1 cup of water for 5 minutes, drain, and mash. Allow to cool. Stir in the yogurt and oil.

APPLICATION Apply this to your face every morning and evening after cleansing.

RICH GIRL EYE CREAM

Avocados contain more protein than any other fruit. Their natural oils offer hydration. Sour cream will lighten dark circles.

1 teaspoon avocado

½ teaspoon sour cream

PREPARATION In a small bowl, mash the avocado with a fork. Blend in the sour cream and mix well.

APPLICATION Massage this gently around the eye area every morning and evening.

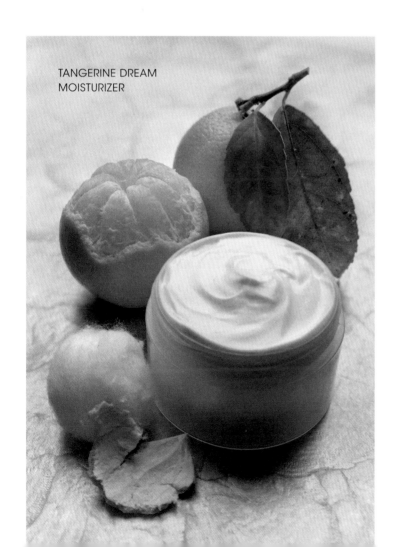

TANGERINE DREAM
MOISTURIZER

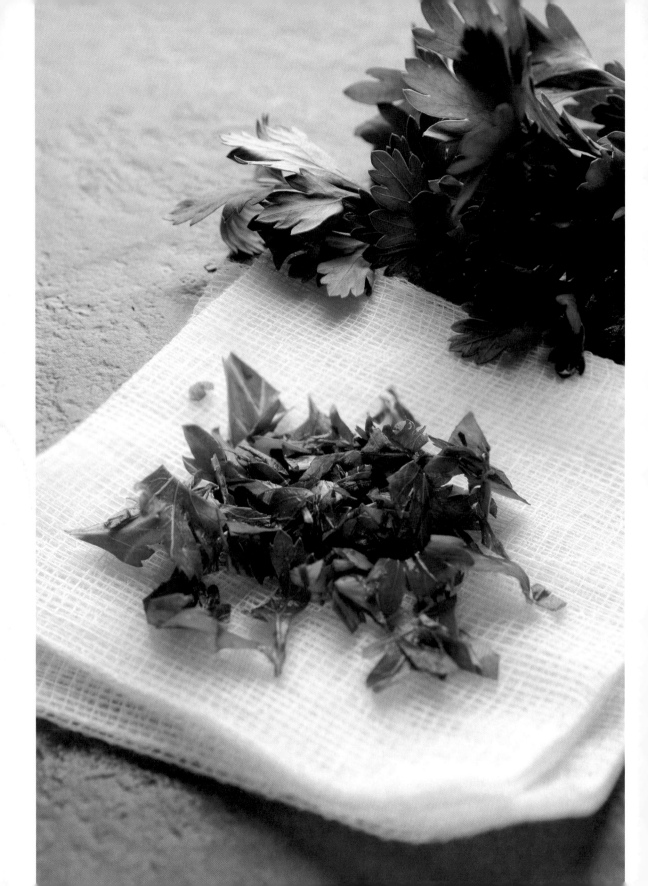

FALL NORMAL-TO-DRY SKIN

Packed away are summer's flip-flops and shorts. It's time for pullovers and boots. In the same way you make adjustments to your wardrobe for the changing weather, you must remember to adjust your skin care regimen.

Plums, flaxseed, and parsley combine with slightly heavier ingredients to create an effortless transition for your skin.

NORMAL-TO-DRY REGIMEN

ALMOND COOL CLEANSER

Almonds act as an anti-inflammatory, antiaging skin tonic that softens, nourishes, and soothes skin.

¼ cup almond milk

2 tablespoons pureed cucumber

1 teaspoon salt

PREPARATION Combine the almond milk, cucumber, and salt in a bowl. Mix well.

APPLICATION Pour a small amount of this onto a clean wet washcloth or sponge. Gently wash your face with this every morning and evening. Rinse off with warm water.

FLAXSEED HEALTHY SKIN CLEANSER

Flaxseed oil contains omega-3 fatty acids, which are highly beneficial to skin. Oatmeal is a gentle skin-softening cleanser. Milk is the ultimate instant skin beautifier.

½ cup warm milk

1 tablespoon oatmeal (old-fashioned, not instant or steel-cut)

1 tablespoon flaxseed oil

PREPARATION In a small microwave-safe bowl, warm the milk in the microwave. Stir the oatmeal into the milk. Add the oil and mix well.

APPLICATION Pour a small amount of this onto a clean wet washcloth or sponge. Gently wash your face with this every morning and evening. Rinse off with warm water.

BLACK PLUM BOUNTIFUL MOISTURIZER

Not only are plums a good source of the antioxidant vitamins A and C, they also contain the important nutrient potassium and fiber. Vegetable oil is a great moisturizer for dry skin.

3 ripe dark plums

1 tablespoon vegetable oil

1 tablespoon sour cream

PREPARATION Skin the plums, then cut them in half and remove the pits. In a food processor or blender, add the plums, oil, and sour cream. Blend until creamy smooth.

APPLICATION Apply this to your face every morning and evening after cleansing. Splash with warm water and pat dry.

CREAMY DATE MOISTURIZER

Dates contain vitamin A, which offers antiaging benefits, and folate, which assists in the production of new skin cells.

3 pitted fresh dates

2 teaspoons cottage cheese

1 teaspoon corn syrup

PREPARATION In a blender, combine the dates, cottage cheese, and corn syrup. Mix well.

APPLICATION Apply this to your face every morning and evening after cleansing. Splash with warm water and pat dry.

MIRACLE PARSLEY HONEY MASK

Parsley is an amazing herb for the face! It can reduce swelling and redness, lighten the skin, even the tone, reduce blackheads, and aid in the prevention of wrinkles. Egg yolk and honey are hydrating tonics for women with drier skin.

2 tablespoons chopped parsley

1 egg yolk

1 tablespoon honey

PREPARATION In a blender, combine the parsley and egg yolk and mix well. Add the honey and mix again.

APPLICATION Apply a thick layer of this to your face and neck and relax for 20 minutes. Rinse off with warm water, then apply your moisturizer.

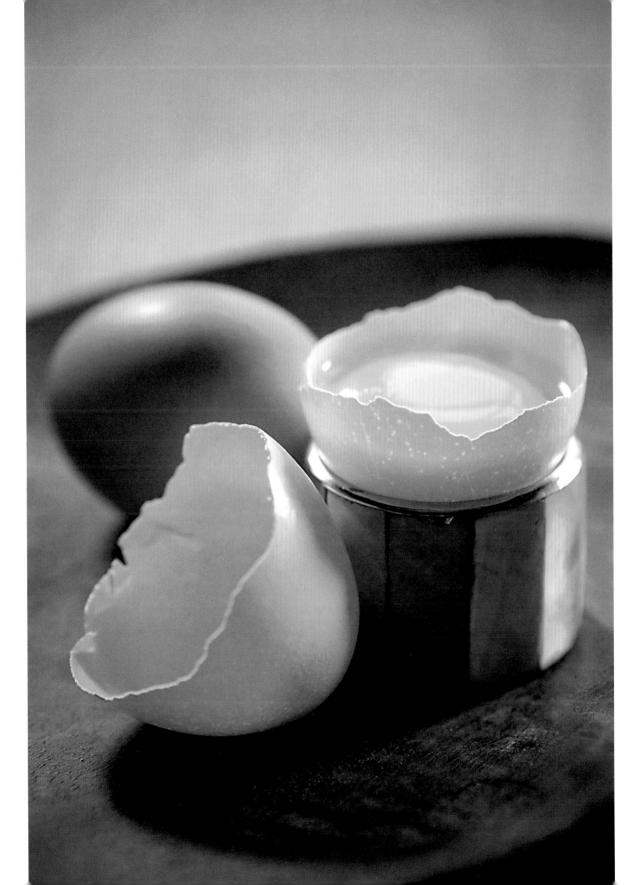

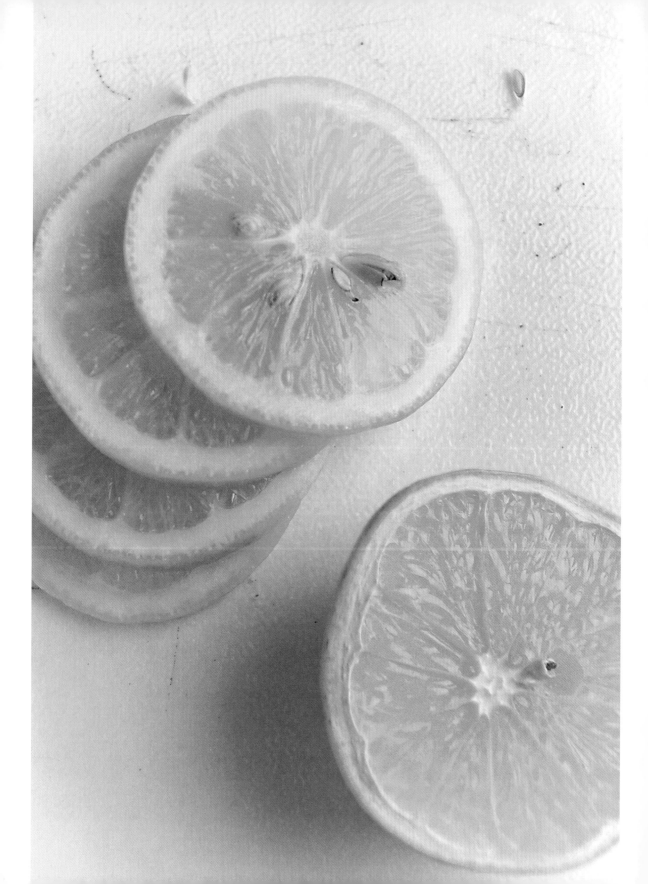

FALL NORMAL-TO-OILY SKIN

Fall is the time for harvesting life's bountiful gifts.
Cantaloupes, lemons, fresh apricots, and kiwis offer special nu-
trients in this season. For normal-to-oily skin, these foods contain
the secret benefits of renewal and rejuvenation.

NORMAL-TO-OILY SKIN REGIMEN

REVITALIZING KIWI CLEANSER

Kiwis contain a high concentration of vitamin C. Their vitamins and minerals gently remove dead skin cells and at the same time reduce the appearance of large pores. Milk detoxifies. Corn oil acts as a natural skin softener.

1 fresh kiwi

¼ cup milk

½ tablespoon corn oil

PREPARATION Peel the kiwi and cut it into several small pieces. In a small microwave-safe bowl, microwave the kiwi for 2 or 3 seconds to soften. In a blender, combine the softened kiwi, milk, and oil. Blend until creamy smooth.

APPLICATION Wash your face with this in the morning and evening. Rinse off with warm water, then rinse with cold water.

JUICY APPLE CLEANSER

Apple juice contains malic acid, which is an excellent exfoliator.

¼ cup apple juice

1 teaspoon baking soda

2 teaspoons plain yogurt

PREPARATION In a blender, combine the apple juice, baking soda, and yogurt. Blend until creamy.

APPLICATION Wash your face with this in the morning and evening. Rinse off with warm water, then rinse with cold water.

GENTLE GIN TONER

Gin has a clean scent and is a natural alcohol that offers gentle tightening for your skin.

2 tablespoons gin

3 tablespoons mineral water

3 tablespoons witch hazel

PREPARATION In a clean plastic bottle, combine the ingredients and shake well.

APPLICATION Wipe this over your face using a clean cotton ball.

SUCCULENT CANTALOUPE COCONUT MASK

Cantaloupe is at its peak in the fall. Juicy and sweet, this fruit is loaded with the important antioxidant beta-carotene. Cantaloupes are also high in vitamin C, and are a good source of potassium and folate.

1 slice cantaloupe

1 tablespoon coconut milk

1 teaspoon almond oil

PREPARATION In a blender, combine the cantaloupe, coconut milk, and oil. Blend until creamy.

APPLICATION Cover your face and neck with a thin layer of this and relax for 20 minutes while enjoying a slice or two of cantaloupe. Rinse off with warm water, then rinse with cold water. Apply your moisturizer.

LEMONY SWEET MOISTURIZER

Lemons whiten and brighten skin without harming the natural oil production.

1 small lemon

1 tablespoon plain yogurt

1 teaspoon vegetable oil

PREPARATION Cut up the lemon, but do not remove the skin. In a blender, combine the lemon, yogurt, and oil. Mix until creamy.

APPLICATION Apply this to your face in the morning and evening after cleansing.

POSITIVELY ENERGIZING GRAPEFRUIT MOISTURIZER

The glorious grapefruit moisturizes skin and prevents wrinkles. Some say it even fights depression—making it a fruit of infectious positive energy! Egg yolk is a natural moisturizer. Honey and butter give you a warm glow. Cottage cheese evens skin tone.

1 tablespoon cottage cheese

½ egg yolk

1 tablespoon honey

1 teaspoon unsalted butter

1 tablespoon grapefruit juice

PREPARATION In a blender or food processor, combine the cottage cheese, egg yolk, honey, and butter. Mix until creamy smooth. Add the grapefruit juice and blend again.

APPLICATION Apply this to your face in the morning and occasionally at night if you feel dry. Your skin type needs only a little bit of moisturizer during this season. Splash with warm water and pat dry.

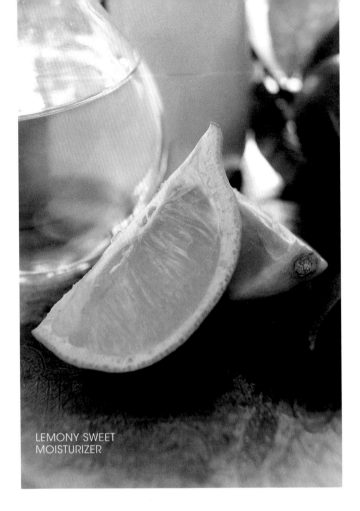

LEMONY SWEET
MOISTURIZER

ALMOND SOFT EYE CREAM

Almond oil is safe to use around the eyes. It can heal even red or irritated skin. Combined with mayonnaise, it perfectly softens to prevent fine lines.

1 tablespoon almond oil

1 tablespoon mayonnaise

PREPARATION In a small bowl, combine the oil and mayonnaise. Mix well.

APPLICATION Gently apply around the eye area.

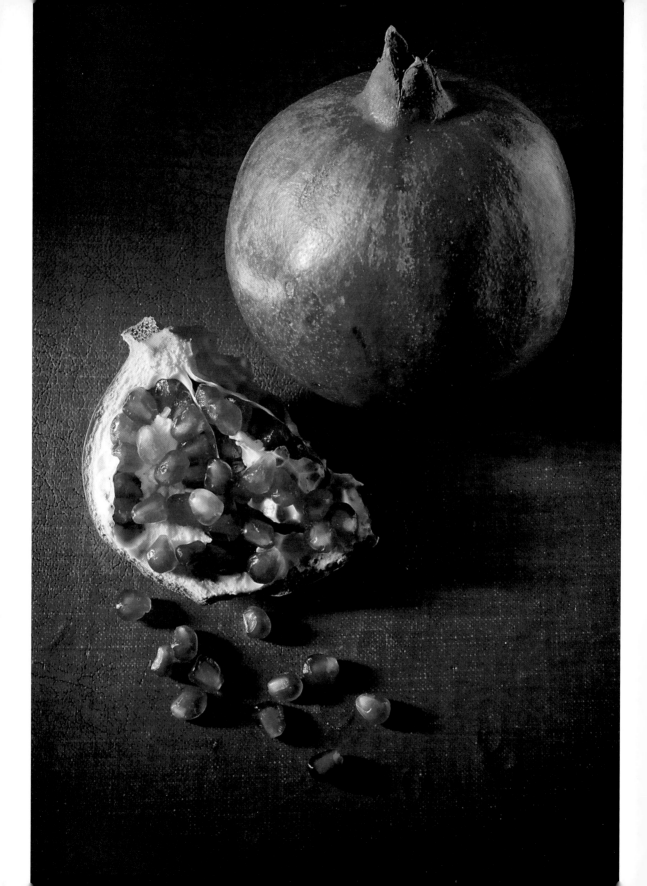

FALL OILY SKIN

The promise of change is in the air and oily skin loves it!

After a hot summer, oily skin must be treated with calming, soothing ingredients that diffuse redness.

Reap the benefits of the healing pomegranate, along with yogurt hydration and tangy tangerine exfoliation.

OILY SKIN REGIMEN

MILKY ROSE CLEANSER

Roses soften and bring a healthy blush to skin. Milk is a soothing skin food.

2 tablespoons chopped rose petals

¼ cup milk

1 teaspoon baking soda

PREPARATION In a blender, combine the petals, milk, and baking soda. Mix well.

APPLICATION Pour a small amount of this onto a clean wet washcloth or sponge. Gently wash your face and neck with this every morning and evening. Rinse with warm water.

GENTLE APPLE OATMEAL CLEANSER

Oatmeal offers gentler cleansing than soap does. Mineral water's high silica content strengthens the cells between the collagen and elastin fibers. Mineral water also plumps the skin and slows the formation of wrinkles. When it's mixed with the toning and softening effects of apple juice, your skin will stay flawless!

1 tablespoon oatmeal (old-fashioned, not instant or steel-cut)

2 tablespoons apple juice

¼ cup mineral water

PREPARATION In a small bowl, combine the oatmeal and apple juice. Slowly add the mineral water to create a thick, creamy mixture.

APPLICATION Pour a small amount of this onto a clean wet washcloth or sponge. Gently wash your face and neck every morning and evening. Rinse with warm water.

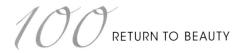

POMEGRANATE POWER TONER

The pomegranate contains more inflammation-fighting antioxidants than red wine or green tea does. Vodka with a pinch of salt removes dead skin cells and acts as an antiseptic for the skin.

3 tablespoons pomegranate juice

¼ cup vodka

½ teaspoon salt

PREPARATION In a clean plastic bottle, combine the pomegranate juice, vodka, and salt. Shake for 30 seconds.

APPLICATION Wipe your face with this as needed, using a clean cotton ball.

TANGY TANGERINE SOUR CREAM MASK

Tangerines are rich in vitamin C. With strong antioxidants, this tasty fruit refreshes and reenergizes skin. Sour cream is added as a wonderful skin softener.

1 large tangerine

1 tablespoon sour cream

PREPARATION Cut the unpeeled tangerine into small pieces. In a food processor or blender, puree the tangerine pieces. Add the sour cream and mix well.

APPLICATION Apply this to your face and neck and relax for 20 minutes. Rinse off with warm water, then apply your moisturizer.

SHINY GOLD MOISTURIZER

Almond oil softens and conditions skin. The citric acid in lemons gently exfoliates dead skin cells.

1 small lemon

1 tablespoon margarine

1 teaspoon almond oil

PREPARATION Peel the lemon and cut it in half. In a small microwave-safe bowl, soften the margarine in the microwave for 2 or 3 seconds. In a blender, combine the lemon, margarine, and oil. Mix until creamy.

APPLICATION Apply this to your face in the morning and evening after cleansing.

FRESH LIME YOGURT MOISTURIZER

Oily skin can use a moisturizer in the fall. Lime juice is overall one of the best foods for your skin. It has rejuvenating powers, effectively prevents blackheads, and gives your face a healthy glow. Lime and yogurt make for a perfect light cream for oily skin.

½ lime

1 tablespoon plain yogurt

1 teaspoon flour

PREPARATION In a blender, combine the lime and yogurt, and mix well. Pour the mixture into a bowl and add the flour. Blend until creamy.

APPLICATION Apply this to your face in the morning and evening after cleansing.

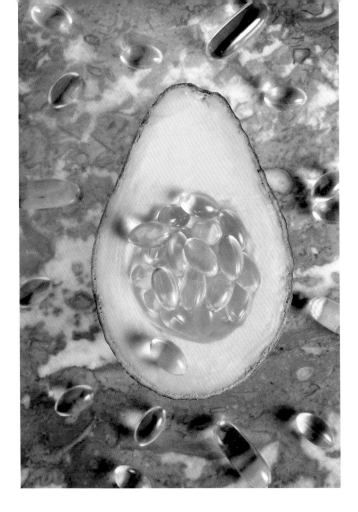

AVOCADO REPAIRING EYE CREAM

Avocados are high in vitamin E. When they are combined with vitamin E oil, you'll have a rich emollient that keeps fine lines at bay. Use sparingly.

1 avocado

3 vitamin E oil capsules

PREPARATION Cut the avocado in half and remove the pit. Scoop out 1 tablespoon of avocado into a small bowl and mash it. Cut off the tips of the capsules. Squeeze the oil onto the avocado and mix well.

APPLICATION Massage a small amount of this gently around the eye area.

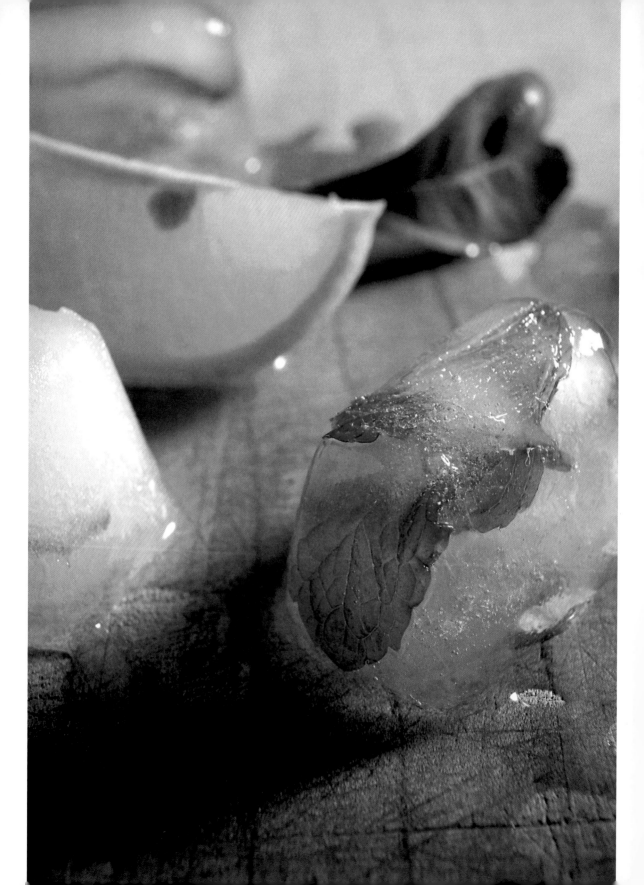

Part 2

SUN SIGNS

According to many ancient traditions, living in rhythm with your sun sign doesn't only offer fun facts about your personality traits and love matches, it also reveals information about your skin's needs. For instance, if you're a Gemini, you must get plenty of rest and relaxation. Cancers require dairy. Leos respond well to figs and coconut. For optimum health, every sign in the zodiac has specific requirements.

The recipes in this section are listed under your element and sun sign. They don't replace your seasonal skin care regimen, but further enhance its effects. By experimenting with these foods, you will discover that everything you are (even your birth date) can play a role in creating your outer (and inner) beauty.

If you have only an hour to get ready, check out the Quick Fix page for your element. There are great tips to keep you looking healthy and delicious!

FIRE ARIES LEO SAGITTARIUS

If you're a fire sign, you were born a leader. You like to make quick, risky, and positive decisions. And you don't like competition! You always want to be first, especially in a beauty contest. You simply must look the best. While this trait can work against you, you could use it for your benefit. Looking beautiful (and feeling it!) helps lead to the fulfillment of your career and life goals.

People love your warm, headstrong, and unruly personality. Best friend matches for you are fellow fire or water signs. Earth and air can dampen your flames.

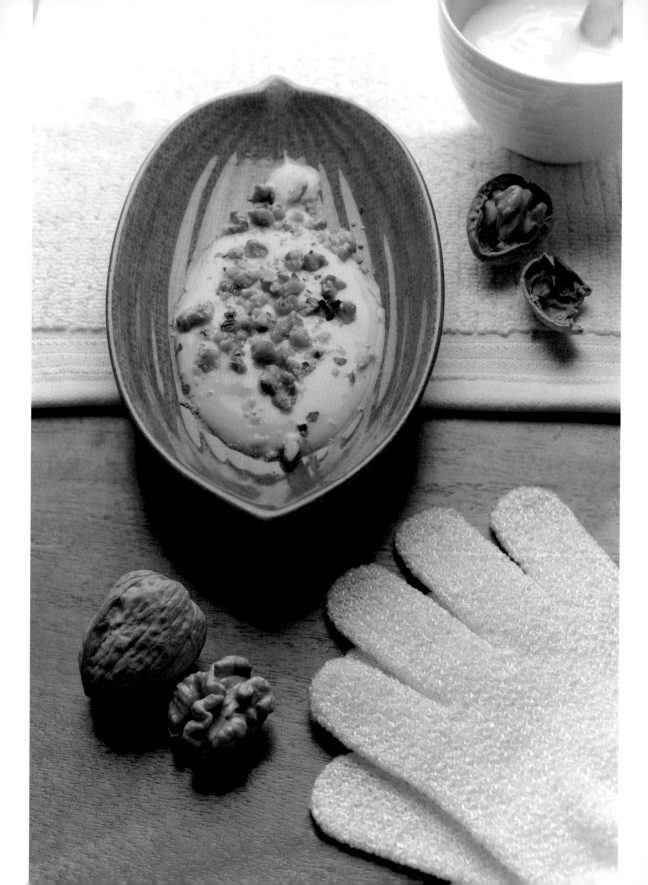

FIRE SIGNS QUICK FIX

After a long day, you come home stressed-out and exhausted. But you can't kick your shoes off and relax just yet—you have an hour to get ready for a dinner party. First thing, calm the flame. Follow these five steps, and you'll soon be back to fabulous!

1. Take a 5-minute shower in warm water. Rinse in cold water for 1 minute.
2. Drink a big glass of cold water or cold orange juice.
3. Soak a soft washcloth in cold water mixed with 1 teaspoon of fresh lemon juice. Leave the compress on your face for 3 to 5 minutes.
4. Make a Quick Fix mask. Mix 2 teaspoons of shredded cucumber with 1 tablespoon of plain yogurt and apply to your face. Cut 2 thin slices of potato and place them over your eyes. Rest for 15 minutes. Rinse off with warm water.
5. Massage a very small amount of mayonnaise over your face for 5 minutes. Mayonnaise contains eggs, vinegar, and lemon, which moisturize, nourish, and restore skin's natural acid levels. Do not rinse off.

Now you are ready to put on your makeup and head out for the dinner party—radiant and refreshed!

ARIES MARCH 21–APRIL 20

> Over the hills and racing through the city—my feet pound to the rhythm of my own heartbeat. I am fire.

Aries carry the most fire. You burn hot day and night. Always on the go, you live your life through your body more than through your mind.

Aries throw all of their energy into everything—especially work. Your aggressive energetic nature, while producing concrete results, can take a toll on your beauty. For this reason, you must get plenty of rest and ingest foods rich in minerals.

BEAUTY TRAITS

Great skin; beautiful facial structure that does not wither with age.

TROUBLE AREAS

Drained energy; sinus trouble; headaches; feet.

FOODS

Broccoli, cucumber, cauliflower, onions, beets, figs, bananas, apricots, pumpkin, beans, swordfish, and veal.

TIPS

When you can remember to, O fiery Aries, take a deep breath. The need to forge ahead doesn't always suit you best.

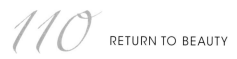

RECIPES

Sit back, relax, and cool down—so that you can go back out and do it all again!

CALM DOWN APRICOT CLEANSER

Apricots are high in iron and great for fixing troubled skin spots. Milk is cooling and soothing, with gentle acidic properties.

1 ripe apricot

½ cup milk

1 teaspoon apple cider vinegar

PREPARATION Peel the apricot and eat the skin, then cut it in half and remove the pit. In a blender, combine the apricot, milk, and vinegar. Blend until smooth.

APPLICATION Gently wash your face in the morning and evening with a small amount of this. Rinse off with warm water.

BE CLEAR-MINDED CUBES

Mint improves concentration and clears the mind.

1 tablespoon lemon juice

5 tablespoons chopped mint

1 cup mineral water

PREPARATION Add the lemon juice and mint to the mineral water. Pour into an ice cube tray and freeze.

APPLICATION In the summertime, or whenever you're overheated, smooth an ice cube over your face.

NUT 'N' HONEY SCRUB

Walnuts are packed with beta-carotene, vitamin E, and alpha-linolenic acid, which helps your skin stay soft, smooth, and supple. Honey assists in sloughing away dead skin cells.

1 teaspoon very finely ground walnuts

1 teaspoon honey

1 teaspoon lemon juice

PREPARATION In a small bowl, combine the walnut powder, honey, and lemon juice. Mix well.

APPLICATION Massage this gently over your face for 5 minutes. Pay attention to your T-zone (chin, nose, and forehead area). Rinse off with warm water.

FIG-ILICIOUS MASK

Figs contain an active enzyme that helps to remove dead cells from the surface of your skin. Bananas contain potassium, which moisturizes and rejuvenates.

3 figs

½ banana

1 tablespoon flaxseed oil

PREPARATION In a blender, mix together the figs, banana, and oil.

APPLICATION Apply this to your face and neck and relax for 20 minutes. Rinse off with warm water.

JUST PLAIN EASY MOISTURIZER

With a clean cotton ball, apply a thin layer of plain yogurt over your face. Do not rinse off.

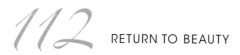

TINGLY TOES FOOTBATH

Mint is a relaxing, cooling, and healing herb.

1 cup fresh mint leaves

4 cups boiling water

2 tablespoons sunflower oil

PREPARATION Chop the mint leaves. Add the mint to the boiling water and steep for 30 minutes. Fill a tub with water for a footbath. Pour the mint water into the tub, then add the sunflower oil.

APPLICATION Soak your feet for 20 minutes, then gently wipe dry with a soft cloth.

MY FEET FEEL GOOD MASK

In the dry cold of winter, this foot mask is relaxing and hydrating.

1 apple, unpeeled

2 cups milk

2 tablespoons jojoba bean oil

PREPARATION Cut the apple into cubes. Cook for 5 minutes in the milk. Mash—do not drain—then add the oil and mix well.

APPLICATION Cover your feet with this mixture, then wrap them in clean gauze. Sit back for 20 minutes and drink a cup of hot mint tea. Unwrap your feet and rinse them with warm water.

LEO JULY 24–AUGUST 23

> Why do I have to give up my dreams?
>
> Why can't I be myself?

Leo, you are the Queen. You love to be admired—and demand to be the only one admired. You respect the finer things in life. Whether it's expensive art, clothing, or a manicure, it's all about looking good. Loving another isn't easy at first, but once you do, you are a loyal and stouthearted friend.

Leos have a secret power. Whatever you believe comes true for you.

BEAUTY TRAITS
Excellent dancer; shiny, thick hair.

TROUBLE AREAS
Heart and back trouble when emotional. The back represents courage; the heart represents your emotions. Take care with simple stretching exercises.

FOODS
Beef, lamb, egg yolks, seafood, whole milk, yogurt, whole wheat, rye, rice, almonds, walnuts, sunflower seeds, beets, asparagus, spinach, raisins, dates, figs, lemons, apples, peaches, coconut, plums, pears, and oranges.

TIPS
Learn to eat healthy meals instead of snacking.
Avoid rich food and wine.
Take short naps for relaxation.
Sunbathe for short periods.

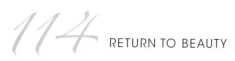

RECIPES

Luxurious desires require fancy recipes!

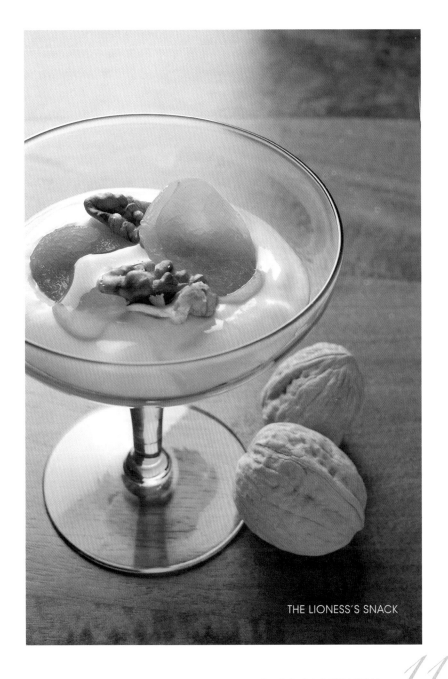

THE LIONESS'S SNACK

MIRACLE APPLE POTATO MASK

Potatoes are packed with vitamin C—an antiaging miracle. Apples bring out a natural glow. Egg yolks are hydrating.

1 small potato, unpeeled, cubed

1 apple, unpeeled, shredded

1 teaspoon olive oil

1 egg yolk

1 tablespoon milk

PREPARATION Cook the potato in 2 cups of water until soft, about 10 minutes. Drain. In a small bowl, mix together the potato, apple, oil, and egg yolk. In a small microwave-safe bowl, warm the milk in the microwave for 2 or 3 seconds. Add the milk and continue to stir until it forms a paste.

APPLICATION Cover your face and neck with this and relax for 20 to 30 minutes. Rinse off with warm water.

DECADENT DÉCOLLETAGE MASK

Move over, Marie Antoinette—this décolletage mask calms the fire in the Lion's breast.

2 teaspoons sunflower oil

1 teaspoon honey

2 teaspoons coconut juice

5 tablespoons sour cream

PREPARATION In a small bowl, mix together the oil, honey, coconut juice, and sour cream.

APPLICATION Gently apply this over your chest and breast area, then lie back and relax for 30 to 40 minutes. Wipe off with a warm washcloth.

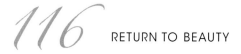

THE LIONESS'S SNACK

Apricots are good for anemia and exhaustion. This snack is the perfect Leo food.

3 tablespoons crushed walnuts

1 tablespoon raisins

6 dried apricots

1 teaspoon lemon juice

4 tablespoons plain yogurt

2 tablespoons honey

PREPARATION In a food processor or blender, mix together the walnuts, raisins, apricots, and lemon juice. Transfer to a bowl and mix with the yogurt and honey.

APPLICATION Eat 1 tablespoon three times a day (after each meal).

SILKY SATIN MANE MASSAGE

Your hair is your thing. Keep it soft and satiny all year long with lemon juice, almond oil, and moisturizing egg yolk. Natural alcohol will make it shine, and will not strip away hair dye.

½ tablespoon lemon juice

2 tablespoons vodka

3 tablespoons almond oil

2 egg yolks

PREPARATION In a small bowl, combine the lemon juice, vodka, oil, and egg yolks. Mix well.

APPLICATION Lean your head back over a sink and pour this onto your scalp. Work it through your hair with your fingertips all the way to the ends. Relax for 20 minutes. Massage your scalp for 10 minutes, then wash with your favorite mild shampoo.

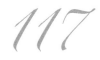

SAGITTARIUS NOVEMBER 23–DECEMBER 22

I wander in search of the truth.

What is the meaning of life and true love?

If you live under Saturn, you mostly have an enthusiastic and positive attitude. When you aren't happy, you hide your tears in your pillow. You love mental exploration. In fact, mental stimulation is a must. You are passionate only about things that are a challenge. Strong and confident, you are the perfect playmate—but only when you're winning. Sagittarians don't take defeat well. If you're unhappy, you won't work on things—you'd rather walk out.

You require minimum care for a healthy life. More octogenarians live under the sign of Sagittarius than any other sign.

Free-spirited and romantic, you believe domestic life equals death. You marry for love, not for money or social standing. When you finally do settle down, you are a delightful companion.

BEAUTY TRAITS
Lean and slender in youth; graceful, well-developed legs; robust health.

TROUBLE AREAS
Hips; liver; poor circulation; dull skin and hair.

FOODS
Boiled fish, fruit and vegetable skin, raw salads, green peppers, figs, prunes, strawberries, pears, apples, potatoes, oats, whole grain cereals, egg yolks, sprouts, beets, tomatoes, asparagus, plums, cherries, skim milk, yogurt, brown rice.

TIPS

Moderate physical activity is a must. If you don't get it, you will get sick. As you
    age, if you're not walking, you will gain weight in your hips and thighs.

Drink a lot of water.

Avoid starches and high-fat foods.

Avoid alcohol, butter, candy, cigarettes, and chocolate.

Avoid sun and wind on your delicate skin.

RECIPES

When you're beautiful, Sagittarius, you shine with confidence!

FRUITY FACE MASK

High in vitamin C, this mask will make you glow!

1 tablespoon shredded apple (unpeeled)

1 tablespoon shredded pear (unpeeled)

1 teaspoon oatmeal (old-fashioned, not instant or steel-cut)

1 teaspoon nonfat milk

PREPARATION In a small bowl, combine the shredded fruits, oatmeal, and milk. Mix
well.

APPLICATION Cover your face and neck with this and relax for 20 minutes. Rinse off
with warm water.

CAESAR SALAD MASK

For Sagittarians prone to oily skin.

5 romaine lettuce leaves, finely chopped

½ teaspoon lime juice

2 teaspoons corn oil

PREPARATION In a blender, mix together the lettuce leaves, lime juice, and corn oil.

APPLICATION Gently cover your face and neck with this and relax for 15 minutes. Rinse off with warm water.

SLEEPY TOES AND FINGERS MASSAGE

This massage will improve your circulation. Don't forget the little things!

2 tablespoons dried chamomile

1 cup milk

1 teaspoon olive oil

PREPARATION In a small saucepan, bring 2 cups of water to a boil, then add the chamomile. Steep for 10 minutes and then strain. Add the milk and allow to cool slightly. Add the olive oil and mix well.

APPLICATION Massage your fingers and toes with this for 15 minutes before going to bed. Wipe off but don't rinse.

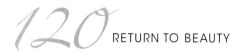

CHEERFUL CHERRY MOISTURIZER

Proven effective in fighting heart disease and inflammatory conditions, the cherry is also regarded as an antiaging fruit in skin care. The egg yolk and cream offer pleasant hydration. Figs are fabulous. Add Cognac, and this moisturizer is perfectly decadent!

2 figs

5 pitted cherries

1 egg yolk

1 tablespoon heavy cream

1 teaspoon Cognac

PREPARATION In a blender, combine the fruits, egg yolk, and cream and mix well. Add the Cognac and blend again until creamy.

APPLICATION Gently cover your face with this in the morning and evening after cleansing. Splash with warm water and pat dry.

THE ARCHER'S MASK

These three ingredients hit the bull's-eye every time as perfect foods for Sagittarian skin care.

1 tablespoon avocado

1 egg yolk

1 teaspoon honey

PREPARATION In a small bowl, combine the ingredients and mix well.

APPLICATION Cover your face and neck with this and relax for 20 minutes. Rinse off with warm water.

EARTH TAURUS CAPRICORN VIRGO

If your sun sign is the element earth, you were born with a natural beauty. You rarely feel insecure, and are stable and well organized. Working is a pleasure for those living on the ground. But sometimes, you can work too hard.

Best friend matches for your element are fellow earth or water signs.

You don't like bright colors or strong scents. You prefer to stay low-maintenance in the self-care department. You always look adorable!

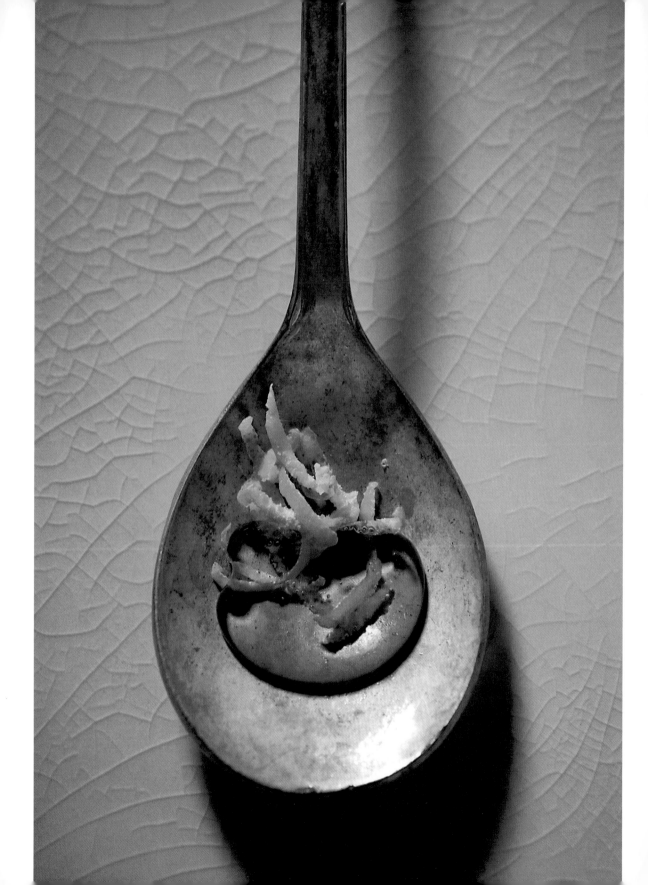

EARTH SIGNS QUICK FIX

Confident that it doesn't take a lot of time for you to get pretty for a big night on the town, after work, you stop to smell the roses. Why not buy some to take home? Flowers, on any occasion, relax those orbiting in the element earth.

1. After you've put the flowers in a vase on the coffee table, eat some grapes (frozen are even more delicious!). You're a hard worker. Grapes are the perfect food for renewing your energy.
2. Soak a washcloth in warm milk. Relax with the compress on your face for 15 minutes.
3. Create a mask with 1 egg yolk, 1 teaspoon of honey, and 2 teaspoons of orange or apple juice. Mix the ingredients together well, then apply to your face.
4. Take 2 clean cotton balls and put a small amount of cottage cheese on each. Place the cotton balls over your eyes and relax for 15 minutes.
5. Rinse your face with warm water. Apply your moisturizer, then add a little makeup.

Once again, you are rosy and glowing. Don't forget to put a flower in your hair as you skip out for the evening!

TAURUS APRIL 21–MAY 21

When I realize I am close to the earth, inner peace fills me.

Taureans live with their minds more than their bodies. You usually have a job that taxes your brain. And you use your eyes a lot at work, so they get puffy. Because you want the best for others, when things don't work out, you often come home drained.

Remember that you are feminine and beautiful, Taurus. You were born smart. You like nice things and have very good taste, especially in music and jewelry. A good friend, you are very loving and giving.

Because you're always mentally active, you must learn to relax and get back inside your body.

BEAUTY TRAITS

Beautiful neck, lovely skin; gorgeous bone structure; beautiful speaking voice.

TROUBLE AREAS

Throat, neck, eyes, facial muscles.

FOODS

Unlike those under other signs, you can eat almost anything you want, as long as it's organic. Incorporate a lot of greens, cucumbers, raw nuts, and pumpkin into your diet.

TIPS

Whatever you eat shows up on your face.
You must eat a lot of healthy foods rich in minerals to perform well at work.
Enjoy sensual foods, like cherries and cranberries, to your heart's content.
Take care in winter to wear a scarf and cover your neck and ears.

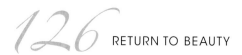

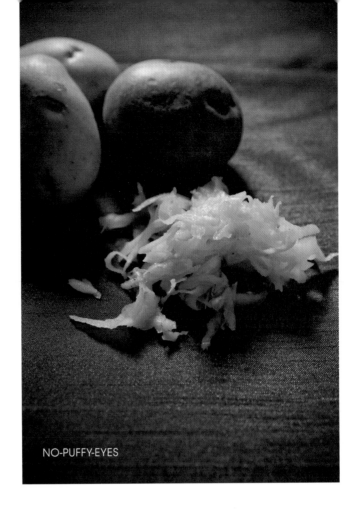

NO-PUFFY-EYES

RECIPES

These recipes were created to calm your mind after another one of your hectic days. Relax and enjoy!

NO-PUFFY-EYES

A little potassium will hide even the most sleepless nights from under your eyes.

1 small potato

PREPARATION Shred the potato, then wrap it in a small piece of gauze.

APPLICATION Put this over your eyes and rest for 15 minutes. Rinse with warm water, then apply your night eye cream.

CREAMY PUMPKIN SPA MASK

Pumpkins are high in vitamins A and C (antioxidants) and zinc—great for the skin.

1 small pumpkin

1 cup warm milk

½ cup mineral water

PREPARATION Halve the pumpkin and peel it. In a small saucepan over low heat, cook the pumpkin in the milk for 30 minutes. Allow it to cool, then cut the pumpkin into very thin slices.

APPLICATION Cover your face and neck with the pumpkin slices and relax for 20 minutes. Rinse with the warm milk, then rinse with the mineral water.

DÉCOLLETAGE BERRY MASK

To ground yourself inside your body, try this sensual, delicious mask.

1 tablespoon cranberries

1 tablespoon blueberries

1 tablespoon yogurt

1 egg yolk

PREPARATION In a food processor, puree the berries. Transfer to a small bowl, add the yogurt and egg yolk, and blend until creamy.

APPLICATION Gently massage this over your breast and chest area. Rest for 20 minutes as you savor a cup of mind-relaxing tea. Rinse off with warm water.

MIND RELAX 'N' REST TEA

Saffron is known to be an excellent stimulator. Taureans love its unique flavor.

1 tablespoon cranberries

¼ teaspoon saffron

PREPARATION In a small saucepan, bring the cranberries, saffron, and 1 cup of water to a slow boil. Simmer for 15 minutes, then strain. Sip and enjoy.

TAURUS REPLENISHING SNACK

Beets are so good for you, Taurus! They are high in fiber, vitamin C, and minerals. Perfect for your tender digestive tract!

2 beets

1 tablespoon ground walnuts

1 tablespoon sour cream

1 teaspoon olive oil

Sea salt

PREPARATION Wash the beets and cook in 4 cups of water for 30 minutes. Drain. Allow to cool, then peel and slice. Transfer to a small bowl, and stir in the walnuts, sour cream, and oil. Salt to taste. Enjoy!

CAPRICORN DECEMBER 22–JANUARY 20

If you can make me laugh, I will give you a happy life.

I am the most womanly of all women.

Capricorns blossom under compliments. In order to thrive, you must be cherished and understood. Because you are prone to introspection and moodiness, it's important to keep your spirits up. You will always stand by those you love.

Grounded and organized, you are excellent with money. Security, both material and financial, is crucial to your state of mind. Even though you may be shy and submissive in appearance, you are the most self-disciplined of all the signs. Self-control is the issue for you.

You love to live in the world. You don't care about trends in fashion or makeup. You know you look good. Yours is a simple, clean beauty. (P.S. You don't like housework.)

BEAUTY TRAITS
Beautiful bone structure, striking; photogenic; health improves with age; known for a long life span.

TROUBLE AREAS
Knees, joints, bones, teeth.

FOODS
A high-protein, high-calcium diet; fresh raw salads and fruit every day; grapes, lemons, figs, celery, cabbage, kale, dandelion greens, spinach, broccoli, corn, peas, potatoes, walnuts, almonds, brown rice, fish, eggs, whole grain bread, cheese, buttermilk, yogurt.

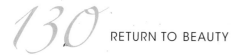

TIPS

Capricorns tend to eat the same foods every day. This can cause a deficiency of
   vitamins in your diet. Be certain to eat a variety of good foods, and don't skip
   meals.

Chocolate and sugar are bad for your skin.

Avoid the sun.

Stay warm and well cloaked in cold, damp weather.

Avoid spicy and overly seasoned foods.

Stretch your spine.

Take good long walks for relaxation.

RECIPES

Here are some recipes to keep your simple beauty simply beautiful.

LIGHT LEMON CLEANSER

*Lemon juice balances the tone of your skin. Eggs yolks are perfect for hydration. Dairy gently
exfoliates dead skin cells without irritating skin.*

1 egg yolk

1 teaspoon sour cream

1 teaspoon fresh lemon juice

1 tablespoon vodka

PREPARATION In a blender, combine the ingredients and mix well.

APPLICATION Wash your face with this every morning and evening.

JUICY HONEY ORANGE MOISTURIZER

The juice makes skin glow. Honey and yogurt hydrate and rejuvenate.

1 tablespoon plain yogurt

1 teaspoon freshly squeezed orange juice

½ teaspoon honey

PREPARATION In a small bowl, combine the ingredients and mix well.

APPLICATION Gently apply this every morning and evening after cleaning.

PERFECTLY PARSLEY MASK

If you have sensitive skin, use this mask three times a week until the problem clears. Parsley is a healing herb. It will even out any discoloration in your skin tone.

4 tablespoons chopped parsley

1 cup warm milk

½ teaspoon cornstarch

PREPARATION Take a clean piece of gauze and cut out holes for your eyes and mouth. In a blender, mix together the parsley, milk, and cornstarch. Soak the gauze in the liquid.

APPLICATION Cover your face and neck with this for 2 minutes, then rinse off with warm water. Repeat two more times.

BETTER BODY BUTTER LOTION

Your beautiful skin will drink in this soothing, rich body lotion.

1 ripe apricot

½ cup buttermilk

1 tablespoon sesame oil

PREPARATION Peel the apricot and remove the pit. In a blender, combine the apricot, buttermilk, and oil. Mix well. Eat the apricot skin—it's high in iron.

APPLICATION Massage this lotion over your body. Pay special attention to sensitive areas such as elbows and knees.

TENDER TOOTH MASK

Because you have sensitive teeth, Capricorn, this mask is a must for you. It will keep your teeth and gums shiny and healthy!

1 teaspoon lemon juice

½ teaspoon baking soda

1 teaspoon bread crumbs

PREPARATION In a small bowl, combine the lemon juice and baking soda. Add the bread crumbs and mash with a fork.

APPLICATION Rub this mask over your teeth with a clean finger, then allow to sit for 10 minutes. Rinse off with warm water.

VIRGO AUGUST 24–SEPTEMBER 23

Still waters run deep!

People often misunderstand those living under the sign of the Virgin. Their first impression of you is often that you are cold and reserved. But living inside you is a reservoir of feeling. You are afraid to trust at first, and you like to be in control of your emotions. Rarely do people realize when you are upset. And you have such nice manners, Virgo, that you rarely complain about your own troubles.

But worry you do. With so many things to think and worry about, you wake up nervous! Frazzled nervous exhaustion makes you the most single girl of all of the signs, because you never take the time to settle down and relax into a relationship.

Loyal and reliable, you are the number one hardworking employee at any company. You love to serve others and prefer that over leadership. You are exacting and hard on yourself, so you must remember to give yourself a break! Find healthy outlets to release your feelings.

You have a great fashion sense, which makes you an excellent trendsetter.

BEAUTY TRAITS
Refined, graceful features.

TROUBLE AREAS
Sensitive nervous system; delicate stomach; ulcers; liver; bowel troubles; eczema, dry skin, and dandruff.

FOODS
Leafy greens, all vegetables, beef, cheese, yogurt, brown rice, oats, corn bread, almonds, oranges, bananas, lemons, melons, apples, pecans, papaya.

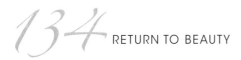

TIPS

Health is a priority for your nerves.

Honey is better for you than sugar.

Chocolate is not good for you, even though you love it! It's too hard on your skin and digestive tract.

Avoid spicy foods.

You don't tolerate medicine well.

RECIPES

You need a little extra help to calm down, emotional Virgo. You must pay attention to whatever you put in, or on, your body.

VIRGO GOOD MORNING

When you awaken in the morning, stretch in bed for a few minutes. Take a deep breath and let it out slowly. Take a quick cold shower to wake up that foggy brain. Don't towel dry—let your skin breathe.

SWEET FACE CLEANSER

Milk is soothing and refreshing as a cleanser. It's good for you to remember to be sweet to yourself every time you wash your face.

¼ cup milk

1 tablespoon baking soda

PREPARATION In a small bowl, combine the milk and baking soda with ½ cup of water. Mix well.

APPLICATION Pour a small amount of this onto a clean wet washcloth or sponge. Gently wash your face, then rinse with warm water.

NICE AND COOL TONER

Because your skin is prone to dryness, lemon and cucumber is the perfect combination.

1 cucumber slice

2 teaspoons vodka

1 teaspoon lemon juice

PREPARATION In a clean container, combine the cucumber, vodka, lemon juice, and ½ cup of water. Shake well and refrigerate for 10 days before using.

APPLICATION Wipe this gently over your face using a clean cotton ball.

LI'L BASIL REJUVENATORS

PREPARATION Chop a small amount of basil and cucumber into small pieces. Mix in water. Pour into an ice cube tray and place in the freezer.

APPLICATION For 1 minute, slide a cube over your face to feel refreshed.

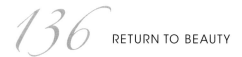

MYSTIC MELON MOISTURIZER

Honeydew melon tones and rejuvenates skin. Butter and egg yolk are hydrating. The honey acts as a gentle exfoliant.

1 tablespoon unsalted butter

1 egg yolk

1 teaspoon honey

1 tablespoon honeydew melon

PREPARATION In a blender, combine the butter, egg yolk, honey, and melon and puree.

APPLICATION While applying your moisturizer, look at yourself in the mirror and repeat: "Nothing can harm me—no wind or sun or rain!" When you're finished, smile—you're ready for your busy day!

ARRIVEDERCI, DANDRUFF

Say good-bye to an itchy, flaky scalp with the magic of apple cider vinegar!

½ cup apple cider vinegar

PREPARATION In a small bowl, combine the vinegar with 1 cup of water.

APPLICATION After shampooing and moisturizing, rinse your hair with this.

VIRGO SWEET DREAMS

1 cup plain yogurt

2 teaspoons honey

PREPARATION In a small bowl, combine the ingredients. Eat before bed to relax and fall fast asleep.

water

WATER

CANCER SCORPIO PISCES

If you're a water baby, you are as pure as clean water. Your facial features are soft and your style is unique—you have great taste!

You work hard to keep everything (and everyone) in harmony and balance. Though it takes a while for you to trust someone, when you do, you're more than happy to let her in on your beauty secrets!

Your best friend matches are fire and earth signs.

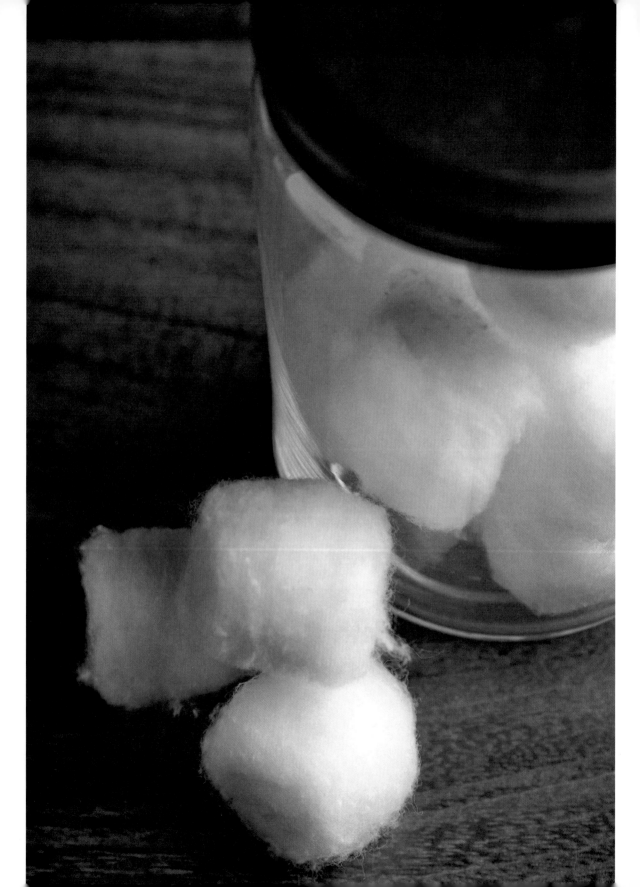

WATER SIGNS QUICK FIX

Sensitive water signs can often get upset during a long day. For this reason, before you go out on your date, you need some extra-tender loving care.

1. When you get home from work, eat 1 or 2 slices of cold cantaloupe or honeydew melon. Melons are a relaxing food.
2. Make the moisturizer recipe for your sign.
3. Now mix 1 teaspoon of salt into 1 cup of warm water. Soak 2 large cotton pads in the mixture.
4. Bring the cotton pads, your moisturizer, 2 cups of milk, 1 cup of plain yogurt, 1 tablespoon of brewer's yeast, a glass, and a spoon into the bathroom. You're going to enjoy a quick-fix spa!
5. Pour the milk into a tub of hot water. Soak for 5 minutes, with the cotton pads on your tired eyes to relax your body.
6. Take a quick cold shower, then pat dry.
7. Fill the glass with hot tap water. Dip the spoon into the hot water. Stand and look at your face in the mirror. (Yes, there may be lines. You may think you look tired.) Using a finger, gently cover the lines with the yogurt. Now take the spoon and gently begin to iron a line in your face, nice and gently. Iron in an upward motion—5 strokes. Dip the spoon into the hot water again and iron another line. Watch the stress instantly disappear from your sweet face!
8. Make a mask by mixing the brewer's yeast with 1 teaspoon of water. Apply the mask. Lie down for 10 minutes or until the mask is dry. Rinse off with warm water, then apply your moisturizer and eye cream. You're ready to put on your makeup.

You are strong and beautiful again! Enjoy your date!

CANCER JUNE 22–JULY 23

With my arms open wide, I lovingly embrace everyone.

Remember that I am sensitive, so please hug back!

If you can coax a Crab to come out of her shell, you will find a nurturing, sensitive, and courageous woman! A Cancer's beauty comes from her generosity. She is very dramatic, and needs love and attention almost as much as vitamins and fresh air.

Cancers can be trusted with your darkest secrets, but they would never trust you with theirs.

She is very sensual and sexual. Everything must be very romantic! If he forgets the flowers and candles, the romance is over!

She always likes to look soft, shy, and innocent. She wants to stay forever young. She never, ever leaves the house with messy hair! Everything must be in its place, whether she's out for a big night or just to pick up milk from the grocery store!

BEAUTY TRAITS
Beautiful, expressive eyes; high cheekbones.

TROUBLE AREAS
Teeth; sensitive skin and stomach.

FOODS
Fish, oysters, egg yolks, milk, yogurt, whole grains, beets, watercress, cheese, lettuce, tomatoes, okra, all fresh fruits.

TIPS
You love sweets, especially chocolate. Remember—eat it in moderation!

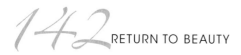

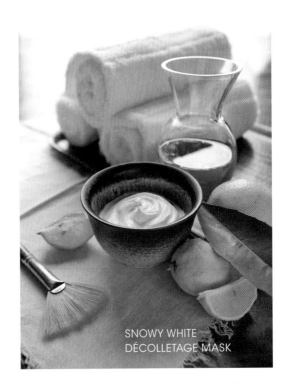

SNOWY WHITE
DÉCOLLETAGE MASK

RECIPES

Your emotions can affect your skin. These recipes will allow you to surrender that hard shell for a moment and enjoy your sensual side!

SNOWY WHITE DÉCOLLETAGE MASK

Dairy is hydrating and soothing, with gentle exfoliating properties. This recipe appeals to your desire to stay forever young. This mask can be done up to three times a week.

2 tablespoons almond milk

1 egg yolk

1 tablespoon fat-free sour cream

PREPARATION In a small bowl, combine the milk, egg yolk, and sour cream and stir until well blended.

APPLICATION Massage this over your breasts and leave on for 10 to 15 minutes. Rinse off with warm water.

APPLES 'N' OATS MASK

Apples tone and renew your skin, leaving it blushing and flawless! Pumpkins contain good nutrition for your face, softening and lightening skin tone. Oats will leave your skin feeling smooth.

2 tablespoons shredded apple

2 tablespoons shredded pumpkin

1 teaspoon flaxseed oil

1 teaspoon oatmeal (old-fashioned, not instant or steel-cut)

PREPARATION In a small bowl, combine the shredded apple and pumpkin. Add the oil and oatmeal and mix well.

APPLICATION Cover your face and neck with this and relax for 10 to 15 minutes. Rinse off with warm water.

SLEEPY SWEETIE TEA

Mint is just the perfect calming herb! Make this tea to take into the bath with you.

1 tablespoon fresh mint leaves

1 teaspoon lemon juice

1 to 2 teaspoons sugar or honey

PREPARATION In a small saucepan, bring 2 cups of water to a boil and add the fresh mint. Steep for 10 minutes, then strain. Add the lemon juice and sugar (or honey, if you prefer) to remove bitterness. Allow to cool. Drink lukewarm.

TIRED-EYES MASK

Lavender is the perfect, calming essential oil. Cucumbers rejuvenate puffy eyes and dark circles. Parsley lightens skin tone.

1 teaspoon lavender oil

1 tablespoon shredded cucumber

1 tablespoon chopped parsley

PREPARATION In a small bowl, mix together the oil, cucumber, and parsley. Carry the bowl into the bathroom to apply during your hot soak.

APPLICATION Pat this over your closed eyes and rest for 10 to 15 minutes. Rinse off with cold water.

NURTURING HOT SOAK

When you're feeling a little too sensitive for the world, climb inside this safe, hot soak and let all your feelings go.

6 tablespoons sea salt

2 tablespoons rose oil

1 teaspoon dry mustard

PREPARATION Into a hot bath, pour the salt, oil, and dry mustard.

APPLICATION Rest for no more than 15 minutes. Rinse off in a cold shower, then a hot shower. Alternate shower water temperature five times.

SCORPIO OCTOBER 24–NOVEMBER 22

Passion, love, and seduction—intensity is everything!

Scorpios are ruled by their sexual drive. You are energetic, imaginative, and passionate. But your passions can lead you into trouble. Without a healthy sex life, your stinger can be biting, dark, and cruel. Brooding is in your nature, but you are also a loyal, non-judgmental, good friend. You're easy to communicate with, even if you never share all of yourself.

When it comes to love, you don't believe in light flirtations, Scorpio. Men can't turn away from your marvelous, fascinating, and irresistible personality. You never have to talk—you say everything with your eyes. Driving men to the brink of insanity, you lift them up to heaven again. Love is all-important to you. No in-betweens. No compromises. You are as entertaining in the living room as you are exciting in the bedroom.

When you are in a good mood, you have the energy of ten women. Scorpios never go halfway on anything! You don't need the last word. You trust your own judgment. Of all the signs, you are the most attentive, emotional, and demanding.

BEAUTY TRAITS

Strong, voluptuous body; beautiful, seductive eyes; excellent recuperative powers; look old in youth, and younger with age.

TROUBLE AREAS

Sinus; when passion is disrupted in any part of your life, it shows up in skin eruptions and urinary tract infections; emotional difficulties that you usually express through sex, if repressed, can cause all forms of illness.

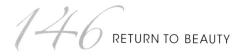

FOODS

Milk, cheese, yogurt, cottage cheese, sprouts, lentils, almonds, walnuts, kale, cucumber, onion, artichokes, Brussels sprouts, tomatoes, watermelon, figs, prunes, black cherries, apples, bananas, pineapples, coconut.

TIPS

Do not eat large meals.

Drink only bottled spring water.

Avoid alcohol.

Take the time for sea travel, the beach, and baths.

Rest.

Flush your system every day with kefir yogurt.

RECIPES

Whether it's the finest Egyptian cotton sheets or the most expensive hotel in Europe, you must be surrounded by the best.

BUTTERY BODY MASK

If your skin is oily or you suffer from eruptions, brewer's yeast is the ultimate nutritional cure.

6 tablespoons brewer's yeast

Buttermilk

PREPARATION Put the yeast into a small bowl. Slowly pour in the buttermilk and stir until the batter is thick and creamy.

APPLICATION Massage this over your breasts and relax for 20 minutes. Rinse off with warm water.

GRACIOUS GRAPEFRUIT MASK

Grapefruit is high in healing vitamin C. It tones and brightens skin, and the citric acid exfoliates dead skin cells.

1 small grapefruit

1 tablespoon honey

1 egg yolk

½ teaspoon flour

PREPARATION Peel the grapefruit. In a blender, combine the grapefruit, honey, egg yolk, and flour. Blend until creamy smooth.

APPLICATION Cover your face and neck with this and relax for 20 minutes. Rinse off with warm water.

SPARKLING STRAWBERRY TONER

Strawberries contain salicylic acid, which removes dead skin cells, leaving your skin bright and healthy.

2 teaspoons chopped strawberries

¼ cup apple cider vinegar

½ cup mineral water

PREPARATION In a blender, combine the strawberries, vinegar, and water. Mix well, then strain.

APPLICATION Smooth this over your face using a clean cotton ball.

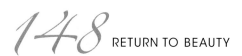

CREAMY COCONUT FACE MASK

Coconut softens, protects, and promotes healing. The lactic acid in milk offers gentle exfoliation.

2 teaspoons shredded coconut

¼ cup milk

1 tablespoon honey

PREPARATION In a small bowl, combine the coconut, milk, and honey. Mix with your hands.

APPLICATION Gently cover your face and neck with this and relax for 20 minutes. Rinse off your hands and face with warm water.

NIGHTTIME EYE REST

Soak cotton balls in milk. Dab gently over your eyes several times before you go to bed.

VOLUPTUOUS VIXEN MASK

Orange zest is packed with vitamin C. It will leave your skin refreshed and smooth. Honey is a luxurious exfoliant.

3 tablespoons orange zest

2 tablespoons honey

1 teaspoon sunflower oil

1 tablespoon freshly squeezed orange juice

PREPARATION In a small bowl, combine the zest, honey, and sunflower oil. Mix well.

APPLICATION Massage this over your breasts. Cover with a clean piece of gauze and relax for 30 minutes. Rinse off with warm water. With a clean cotton ball, dab the orange juice across your breasts. Do not rinse off.

PISCES FEBRUARY 20–MARCH 20

How do I live in the world with so many daydreams and visions?

Pisceans are sensitive to the slightest nuance in their surroundings. You have an affectionate personality that sometimes leads to codependency. Because of your psychic and intuitive nature, you require more patience and sympathy from others. Pisceans can't stand any hint of rejection. Your many moods are like the March wind.

You are caring and affectionate. Your sensual nature shines through as if you were always in the midst of a grand romance.

Graceful and free-spirited, you hate to be boxed in by a boring nine-to-five job. Yearning, always yearning, to fly to the constellations! Fine arts, music, and dance are good career choices for you.

BEAUTY TRAITS

Small feet, fingers, and hands; silky, soft skin; fine hair; graceful, simple beauty. As you age, your dimples deepen, never wrinkle!

TROUBLE AREAS

Health is not robust; you do not easily fight disease; you are vulnerable to cold and sinus troubles; feet; water retention; illnesses can often be emotionally based.

FOOD

Liver, lean beef, lamb, egg yolks, oysters, kidneys, cheese, yogurt, nuts, barley, dried beans, whole grain cereals, beets, spinach, onions, lettuce, raisins, prunes, dates, grapes, peaches, apricots, oranges, lemons, apples.

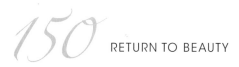

TIPS

Eat a high-protein, low-fat, and low-sugar diet.

Avoid table salt, coffee, and sugar.

Avoid alcohol and drugs, as you are prone to addictions.

Get lots of rest to keep up vitality.

Best exercises for you are swimming and dancing.

Well-fitting shoes are a must.

Never walk with wet feet or sit in a wet swimsuit at the beach or you might catch a cold.

RECIPES

Lucky Pisces, you naturally have beautiful skin. When you take good care of it, it will reward you with beauty for life!

BEAUTIFUL FISHES MASK

(DRY SKIN)

Cabbage and chamomile soothe and hydrate sensitive, dry skin.

1 tablespoon dried chamomile

2 cabbage leaves

2 tablespoons olive oil

PREPARATION In a small saucepan, bring 3 cups of water to a boil. In a small bowl, pour 1 cup of the water over the dried chamomile and steep for 10 minutes. In another small bowl, pour the rest of the hot water over the cabbage leaves. Steep for 1 minute. Pat the leaves dry, then brush them with the olive oil. Strain the chamomile into a separate bowl.

APPLICATION Cover your face and neck with the cabbage leaves and relax for 20 minutes. Rinse off with the chamomile water.

BEAUTIFUL FISHES MASK

(OILY SKIN)

Grapes are great for oily skin! With honey and dairy, they exfoliate dead skin cells, leaving skin smooth and supple. They also keep blemishes at bay.

2 tablespoons cottage cheese

1 tablespoon honey

1 tablespoon red grape juice

PREPARATION In a bowl, combine the cottage cheese, honey, and grape juice. Mix well.

APPLICATION Cover your face and neck with this and relax for 20 minutes. Rinse off with cold water.

MANAGE YOUR MANE MASK

For silky hair, nothing beats the nutrition of hops.

2 tablespoons bread crumbs

1 cup warm beer

PREPARATION In a small bowl, soak the bread crumbs in the beer for 2 hours.

APPLICATION Massage this into your hair and scalp and relax for 45 minutes. Rinse off with Shiny Hair Rinse (opposite).

SHINY HAIR RINSE

You can use this apple cider vinegar rinse once a month for healthy, shiny hair.

4 cups warm water

½ cup apple cider vinegar

PREPARATION In a bowl, combine the water and vinegar.

APPLICATION Pour this over your hair in the shower or over the sink.

JAVA JUICE BODY SCRUB

Rubbing your skin with coffee grounds increases the blood flow and circulation, which is said to facilitate the breakdown of fats beneath the skin, helping to eliminate cellulite.

2 oranges

2 cups plain yogurt

2 tablespoons honey

3 tablespoons coffee grounds

PREPARATION Peel the oranges. In a blender, mix together the oranges, yogurt, and honey. Pour into a bowl, then stir in the coffee grounds.

APPLICATION In the shower, scrub this into your skin with your hands.

AIR GEMINI LIBRA AQUARIUS

Air signs flit and fly through life like beautiful butterflies.

If you are a creature of the air, you are very independent and secure. You feel you are always right, but you usually have nice manners about it. Your best friend matches are fellow air or water signs.

Air signs have a clean beauty, wear very little makeup, and always smell delicious—naturally!

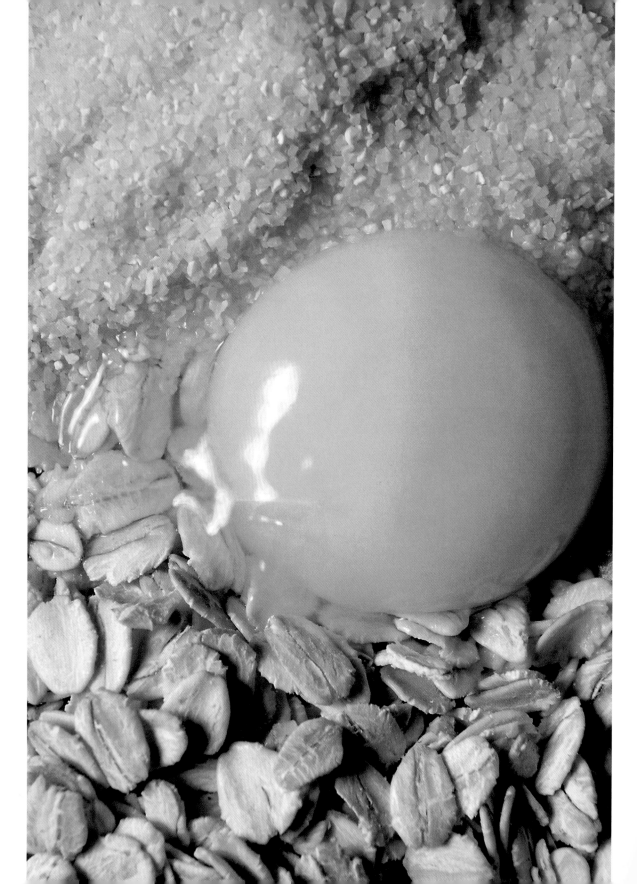

AIR SIGNS QUICK FIX

It's been a long and tiring day at work. All you want is to get home and unwind. Suddenly, you remember that your best friend's art opening is in two hours. Your nervous energy and spinning thoughts need a little soothing. Follow this simple recipe and your anxiety and exhaustion will be transformed into radiant night energy!

1. As soon as you get home, drink a cup of chamomile tea (or a noncaffeinated hot tea of your choice). Eat a banana—potassium is invigorating.
2. For 20 minutes, relax to soothing music. Air signs need music and quiet meditation to stay happy. If you can, make this a 20-minute nap!
3. Move slowly into the kitchen to make a scrub and a mask.

> Scrub: Combine 1 teaspoon of sugar with ½ teaspoon of fresh lemon juice. Mix well.
>
> Mask: In a small bowl, beat 1 egg yolk (for dry skin) or 1 egg white (for oily skin) with 1 tablespoon of honey and 1 teaspoon of oatmeal. Mix well.

4. In a warm shower, mix the scrub in your palm. Massage your face gently with it, paying attention to your chin, nose, and forehead. Clean with soap and water.
5. After drying off, apply the mask to your face, then relax for 15 minutes. While resting, massage your ears. The rim of your ear holds a line of acupressure points that soothe and reenergize. After massaging, pull up on your ears several times, then pull the lobes down several times, then pull the sides of your ears out several times. Doesn't that feel great?
6. Rinse your mask off with water, then apply your moisturizer. You are ready to put on your makeup and take center stage at the art opening.

GEMINI MAY 22–JUNE 21

"Who has the time for a beauty routine with so many important

things on my mind?" she asked her reflection in the clouds.

The Twins flit and fly through life more than any other sign. Your beauty comes from a restless and brilliant mind. People love your charming wit and sparkling personality.

With your beguiling, flirtatious disposition, others may not realize that you are also deeply spiritual, romantic, and altruistic. And there is a hidden dark side you must pay attention to, or it will wreak havoc in your life.

With several personalities, it can be hard to make a decision.

For Gemini women, relaxation is not just something that's nice if you can get it, it is essential to your well-being. You expend a great amount of nervous energy, so you need downtime to rejuvenate.

People rarely see you at the beauty counter!

BEAUTY TRAITS

Graceful neck, shoulders, and arms; beautiful hands.

TROUBLE AREAS

Upper respiratory infections, bronchitis, and asthma.

FOODS

Tomatoes, green beans, spinach, carrots, oranges, peaches, plums, almonds, pomegranates. Calcium-rich foods include dark leafy greens, milk, cheese, yogurt, and cottage cheese.

TIPS

To balance and maintain your energy, Gemini, you must eat a proper diet.
Avoid coffee and cigarettes.

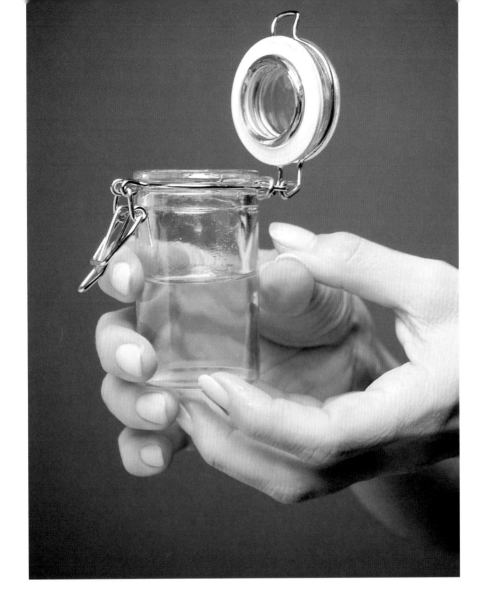

RECIPES

After a long day of thinking "important" things, you need soothing recipes for rejuvenation and relaxation. When stressed, you have a hard time remembering to take deep breaths.

RELAXING POM TEA

Pomegranates are good for the lungs and relax the nervous system. They are also good during menopause.

2 tablespoons pomegranate skin (white)

1 teaspoon honey

PREPARATION In a small saucepan, boil the pomegranate skin with 2 cups of water for 15 minutes. Allow to cool. Strain, then stir in the honey. Sip slowly.

ORANGE CRÈME FACE MASK

Vitamin C and dairy are the perfect foods for Gemini skin. They combine antiaging properties with gentle exfoliation.

2 tablespoons cottage cheese

¼ cup orange juice

½ teaspoon cornstarch

PREPARATION In a small bowl, mix together the cottage cheese and orange juice. Add the cornstarch and mix well. Soak gauze in the mixture.

APPLICATION Lie back with the gauze covering your face and neck and relax for 20 minutes. Rinse off with warm water.

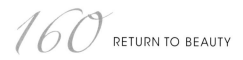

SOOTHING PUMPKIN APRICOT MOISTURIZER

1 slice pumpkin

½ teaspoon baking soda

1 tablespoon apricot kernel oil

½ tablespoon distilled water

PREPARATION Peel and cube the pumpkin. Boil the pumpkin in 1 cup of water for 5 to 7 minutes to soften it. Drain. In a blender or food processor, combine 3 tablespoons pumpkin with the baking soda, oil, and water and mix well. Pour into a small microwave-safe bowl and heat on high for 20 seconds. Allow to cool. Refrigerate in a clean plastic container for up to 1 week.

APPLICATION Gently apply this to your face every morning and evening after cleansing.

GRACEFUL HANDS MASK

Gemini women are renowned for their graceful hands. This mask will keep your hands soft and supple.

1 tablespoon warm milk

2 egg yolks

1 tablespoon honey

1 teaspoon dried chamomile

1 teaspoon rose oil

PREPARATION In a small bowl, combine the ingredients and mix well.

APPLICATION Massage and rub this over your hands. Cover for 20 minutes, then rinse off with warm water.

Up and down. Up and down.

I need a little pampering, to get back to my center again.

Librans, you crave beauty—whether it's food or art or decorating the perfect home. You must be surrounded by flowers and music all the time. Unsure of your feelings, you ride the seesaw of life's ups and downs.

Librans are in love with the idea of love. Enchanting men is your art form. You move like a prima ballerina through their lives.

Libra, you must maintain balance in every area of your life—relationships, work, playtime, exercise, and diet—in order to function to the best of your ability.

BEAUTY TRAITS

Graceful curvature of the spine and lower back; beautiful derriere; fine sensitive skin with pleasing features; good bone structure; high energy level.

TROUBLE AREAS

Skin; hair; throat; kidneys; cold hands and feet; circulation. If there is any inner imbalance or disagreement in your life, your lower back is the first to notice.

FOODS

Fish, poultry, very little beef or lamb, strawberries, apples, raisins, almonds, asparagus, corn, carrots, spinach, beets, tomatoes, wheat, brown rice.

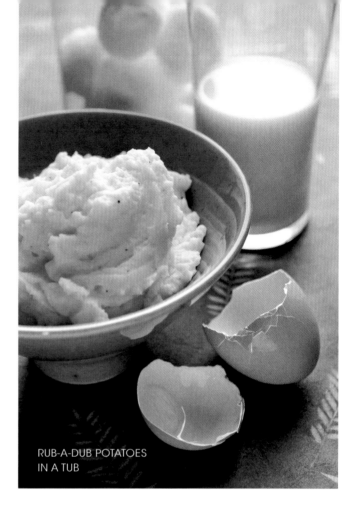
RUB-A-DUB POTATOES
IN A TUB

TIPS

Eat a high-protein, low-fat diet.

You must drink a lot of water.

Avoid carbonated beverages.

Mild exercise is best.

Rich foods, too much champagne, and lack of sleep are your downfalls.

Relax your emotions and your mind!

RECIPES

To keep yourself healthy and in balance, the first thing you love to do is pamper yourself with a facial.

SIMPLY STRAWBERRIES FACE MASK

Vitamin C, from the strawberries, is great for energy, even skin energy. Egg whites tighten skin. Honey acts as a natural exfoliant. Combined, these ingredients bring harmony.

1 egg white

1 tablespoon mashed fresh strawberries

1 teaspoon honey

PREPARATION Whisk the egg white. In a blender, combine the strawberries, egg white, and honey. Mix well.

APPLICATION Gently cover your face and neck with this and relax for 20 minutes. Rinse off with cold water.

JUICY 'N' ORANGEY MASK

(If fresh strawberries are out of season)

Beta-carotene is the nicest thing you can do for yourself. This mask is great for helping fine lines disappear. Drink the extra fresh juice while you relax with this reenergizing mask.

3 teaspoons carrot juice

2 tablespoons cottage cheese

PREPARATION In a blender, mix together the carrot juice and cottage cheese.

APPLICATION Gently cover your face with this and relax for 30 minutes. Rinse off with warm water.

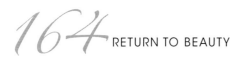

RUB-A-DUB POTATOES IN A TUB

This hand-and-foot duo is perfect in cold weather—and great for circulation!

FEET PREPARATION

Boil 2 cubed potatoes in 6 cups of water for 30 minutes. Remove the potatoes and set aside. Pour the water into a foot tub. Add ½ teaspoon of baking soda and 1 tablespoon of olive oil.

HAND PREPARATION

In a small bowl, mash the potatoes. Add 1 tablespoon of warm milk.

FEET APPLICATION

Sink your feet into the heavenly warm potato water.

HAND APPLICATION

Cover your hands with the mashed potato mixture, then cover them with clean gauze.

FINALE

Relax for 20 minutes, then rinse off your hands and feet in warm water. Rub vitamin E oil into your feet and wear socks to bed. Sleep tight!

LOVELY LIBRA LIGHT DINNER

Libras shouldn't eat big meals or ingest rich food—especially at night.

2 cups cubed watermelon

½ cup feta cheese

Chopped fresh mint

In a bowl, combine the watermelon and cheese. Sprinkle with fresh mint to taste.

AQUARIUS JANUARY 21–FEBRUARY 19

There's so much to be discovered in the world.

Nothing can stop me!

Aquarius, you are the liberated woman of the women's liberation movement—independent, progressive, and forward-thinking. You love to throw your imagination and ideas into social issues. Helping others is a lifelong passion. Though you need a little quiet time to regroup, you can be prone to depression when you spend too much time alone.

Aquarians have a special magnetism. Because you live in the world of ideas, you embody an alluring and distant glamour that men just can't resist. A warm, vibrant romantic streak runs through your veins; however, you are more comfortable with rationality. Be sure to let your guard down when you want love to enter your life. Communication is more important to you than passion. You are an unconventional lover—never jealous, unreasonable, or clinging—and this makes you the perfect mate.

BEAUTY TRAITS
Strong, healthy immune system; well-shaped legs and slender ankles.

TROUBLE AREAS
Circulatory system; ankles, calves, and lower legs; tendency to put on weight if you're not careful; dramatic changes in health; varicose veins and leg cramps; anemia; cold weather is hard on you; headaches; premature gray hair.

FOODS
Ocean fish, lobster, tuna, clams, oysters, beef, chicken, veal, yogurt, cheese, broccoli, carrots, peppers, tomatoes, spinach, radishes, celery, cabbage, lettuce, corn, squash, lentils, almonds, pecans, pears, apples, peaches, lemons, oranges.

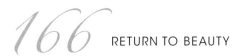

TIPS

Aquarians tend to skip well-balanced meals in favor of snacks. You must eat well-balanced meals.

Limit fat intake. A high-protein diet is best.

Avoid coffee.

Enjoy fresh air and exercise.

Elevate your legs every night for 20 minutes.

Eat plenty of foods high in vitamin C for good circulation in your legs.

RECIPES

Because you love to snack, below is a quick one-week diet to break the bad cycle.

BREAKFAST

1 cup of low-fat cottage cheese with 2 tablespoons of crushed pineapple

LUNCH

1 piece of broiled chicken or fish with 1 cup of cooked spinach or a grilled portobello mushroom marinated in olive oil, soy mayo, salt, and pepper, on a toasted bun with lettuce, tomato, and onion. Serve with sliced avocado.

DINNER

1 piece of steak no bigger than your palm, broiled or grilled, or grill 1 slice of firm tofu marinated in equal parts honey and orange juice (plus some minced garlic). Serve with 1 cup of steamed veggies of your choice and wild rice pilaf. Enjoy an orange for dessert.

To help satisfy your cravings, you can eat 1 cup of cooked oatmeal with 1 piece of dark chocolate as an after-dinner snack.

YUM-YUM MASK

Pears are rich in vitamins C and K, which aid in healing bruises and dark circles. Apples contain iron, which is good for Aquarians who suffer from anemia. Coconuts soften, protect, and promote healing.

1 tablespoon shredded pear (unpeeled)

1 teaspoon shredded apple (unpeeled)

1 teaspoon shredded coconut

1 teaspoon plain yogurt

PREPARATION In a small bowl, combine the fruit and yogurt. Mix well.

APPLICATION Liberally cover your face and neck with this and relax for 20 minutes. Rinse off with warm water. Yes, you can lick this delicious mask off your fingers!

C-BEAUTY TONER

It's all about vitamin C! Vodka is a natural alcohol that helps close pores. Witch hazel is a healing astringent.

¼ cup orange juice

2 teaspoons vodka

2 teaspoons witch hazel

PREPARATION In a clean plastic bottle, combine the ingredients and shake until well mixed.

APPLICATION Wipe your face in the morning and at night with this, using a clean cotton ball.

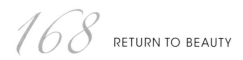

SKIN-SOFTENING DÉCOLLETAGE MASK

This mask softens and adds elasticity to your skin.

2 egg yolks

¼ cup beer

PREPARATION In a small bowl, mix the egg yolks and beer. Soak clean cotton balls in the mixture for several minutes.

APPLICATION Dab the cotton balls over your breasts and chest and relax for 20 minutes. Rinse off with warm water.

THE WATER CARRIER LEG SOAK

1 tablespoon sea salt

1 tablespoon dry mustard

Mix the ingredients into hot water in a foot tub. Soak your calves and ankles for 20 minutes.

HEADACHE THERAPY

Hard-boil 2 eggs; do not peel. When they are cool to the touch, roll the eggs over your forehead and eyebrow area. Practice relaxing your face muscles.

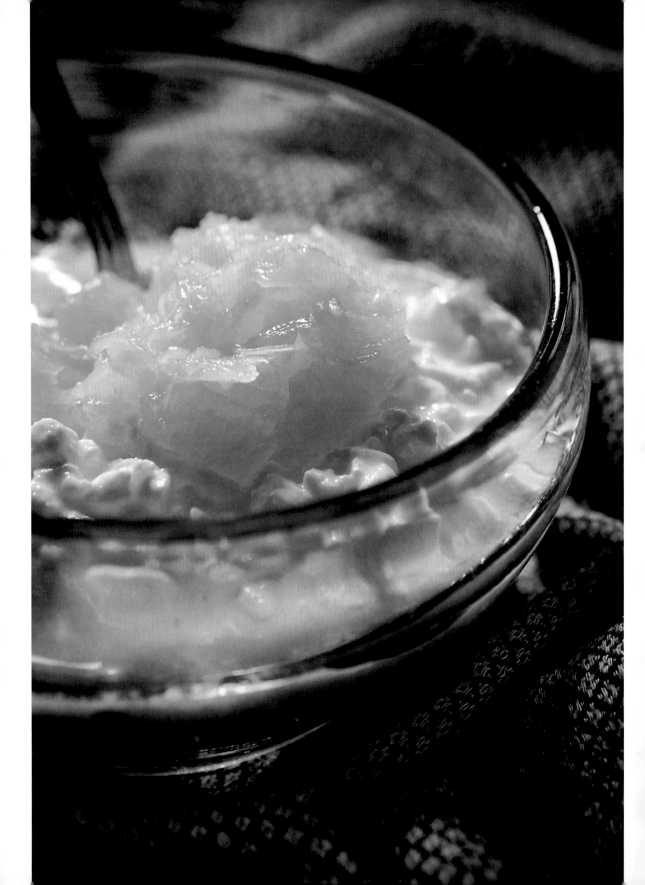

Part 3

SIMPLE SOLUTIONS

It may be the twenty-first century, but old-world wisdom still works best when you have a beauty issue that needs a quick resolution.

From the top of your head to the tips of your toes, these recipes offer solutions that work when you need them!

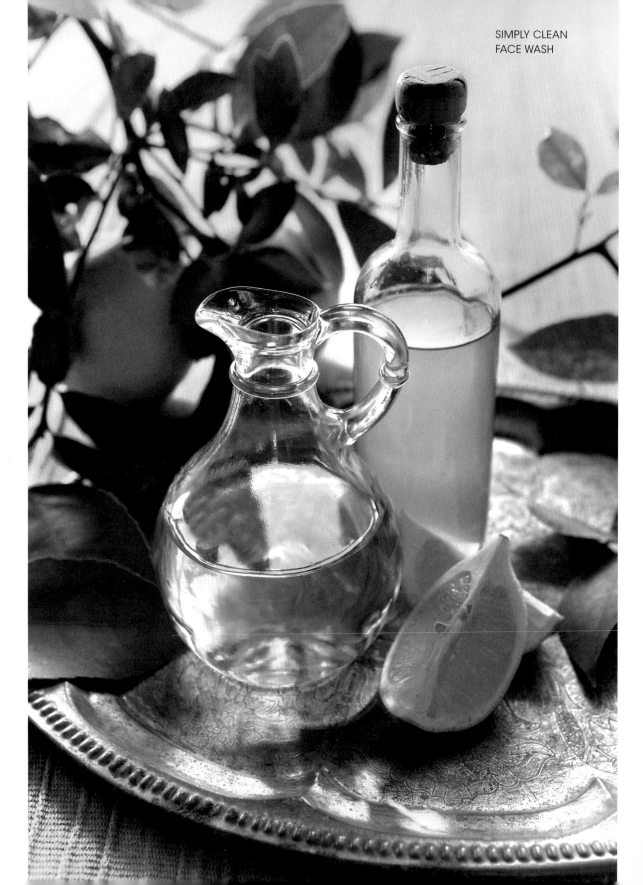

BREAKOUTS, PIMPLES, AND ACNE

If you're having a hard time with breakouts, pimples, or acne, use this safe, natural wash until your skin clears.

SIMPLY CLEAN FACE WASH

Baking soda enhances the citric acid properties of lemon juice—helping to clean and then close your pores.

¼ cup warm water

1 teaspoon baking soda

1 teaspoon lemon juice

PREPARATION In a small bowl, combine the ingredients.

APPLICATION Pour a small amount of this onto a clean wet washcloth or sponge. Gently wash your face, then rinse with warm water.

SPOT TREATMENT

For pimples, smash a little fresh onion and dab it on the spot.

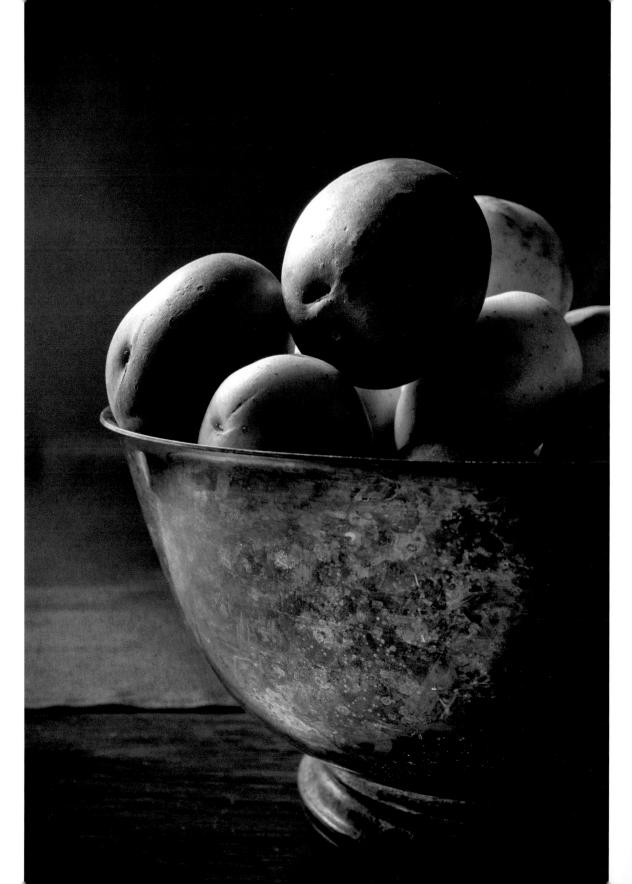

FINE LINES AND WRINKLES

Throughout history, women have fought the signs of aging. Everyone wants to stay attractive and desirable, no matter her age. But real beauty doesn't have a timeline. I've known young women who were physically pretty but lacked any real inner beauty, and elderly women who shone with grace and dignity!

The lines on your face are a map of your life. Unless you want plastic surgery, they are not going to disappear. These mask recipes will keep your skin soft and supple. There are things you can do as well to minimize the appearance of fine lines and wrinkles.

1. Too much time in the sun causes real skin damage, which shows up later in your life as deep lines or, worse, melanoma. When we were young, sometimes we forgot to use sunscreen. Now use a good one!
2. Remember to wash and moisturize your face.
3. Eat right and get plenty of rest.
4. Other things that age us are stress, worry, anger, and other intense emotions. You are in control of your feelings. Think good thoughts. Enjoy grand adventures. Do you want smile lines or frown lines? Remember to laugh!

This life is beautiful—but it is also very short. Don't waste it worrying about getting older. When you take good care of yourself, at any age, the first impressions you give others are of self-confidence and love.

FOR FINE LINES

Depending on your skin type, your lifestyle, and the climate you live in, fine lines can begin to appear even in your late twenties. These recipes contain hydrating foods that will give you a more youthful appearance, and keep those wrinkles from showing up too soon!

JUICY AND CREAMY MASK

1 teaspoon dried chamomile

1 teaspoon carrot juice

2 teaspoons sour cream

1 egg yolk

PREPARATION In a small saucepan, bring the dried chamomile and 1 cup of water to a boil. Steep for 10 minutes, then strain and set aside. In a small bowl, mix together the carrot juice and sour cream. Stir in the egg yolk and mix well.

APPLICATION Gently apply this over your face and relax for 30 minutes. Wash it off with the cooled chamomile tea.

ITALIAN BREAKFAST MASK

2 teaspoons oatmeal (old-fashioned, not instant or steel-cut)

5 teaspoons warm milk

1 teaspoon olive oil

PREPARATION In a small bowl, combine the oatmeal and milk. Add the olive oil and mix well.

APPLICATION Gently apply this over your face and relax for 15 minutes. Rinse off with warm water.

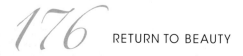

STRAWBERRY FLOWER MASK

1 teaspoon dried lavender

6 ripe strawberries

1 teaspoon corn oil

1 teaspoon honey

½ cup cold milk

PREPARATION In a small saucepan, bring the dried lavender and 1 cup of water to a boil. Steep for 10 minutes, then strain. In a small bowl, mash the strawberries. Add the oil, honey, and lavender extract. Mix well.

APPLICATION Gently apply this over your face and relax for 15 to 20 minutes. Dipping a clean cotton ball into the cold milk, gently wipe off the mask.

PURIFYING YOGURT MASK

1 teaspoon dried chamomile

1 small onion

1 teaspoon plain yogurt

1 egg yolk

1 teaspoon honey

PREPARATION In a small saucepan, bring the dried chamomile and 1 cup of water to a boil. Steep for 10 minutes, then strain and set aside. In a food processor or blender, combine the rest of the ingredients.

APPLICATION Gently apply this over your face and relax for 15 to 20 minutes. Rinse off with the chamomile tea.

ROSY GLOW MASK

1 small apple, unpeeled

1 teaspoon olive oil

1 teaspoon milk

1 egg yolk

PREPARATION Shred the apple. In a small bowl, combine the oil, milk, and egg yolk. Add the apple and mix well.

APPLICATION Gently pat this over your face and relax for 20 minutes. Rinse off with warm water.

EDIBLE PEAR MASK

1 small pear

1 egg yolk

1 teaspoon honey

1 teaspoon flour

PREPARATION Peel the pear and cut it in half. Remove the seeds and cut the pear into cubes. Boil the pear in 1 cup of water for 5 to 7 minutes. In a small bowl, mash the pear, then add the egg yolk, honey, and flour and mix well.

APPLICATION Gently pat this over your face and relax for 20 to 30 minutes. Rinse off with warm water.

POTATO PANCAKE MASK

1 medium potato

2 teaspoons flour

2 teaspoons warm milk

PREPARATION Peel and shred the potato. In a small bowl, combine the flour and milk, then add the shredded potato.

APPLICATION Gently pat this over your face and relax for 10 to 15 minutes. Rinse off with cold water.

COOL MELON MASK

1 slice honeydew melon

1 tablespoon milk

1 teaspoon honey

PREPARATION In a food processor or blender, combine the ingredients.

APPLICATION Gently apply this over your face and relax for 20 minutes. Rinse off with warm water.

ZUCCHINI MASK

1 small zucchini

1 teaspoon flour

PREPARATION Shred the zucchini (do not peel it). In a small bowl, mix the zucchini with the flour.

APPLICATION Cover your face with this mixture, then cover with clean gauze and relax for 15 to 20 minutes. Rinse off with warm water.

TEA TREATMENT

1. Mix ½ cup of water and ½ cup of warm milk.
2. Dip a clean cotton ball in the mixture and cover your face with it. Do not rinse off. Save the milk water to use again at the end of the treatment.
3. Make this mask:

>   1 teaspoon dried black tea
>
>   1 teaspoon mayonnaise
>
>   1 teaspoon sour cream
>
>   1 teaspoon vegetable oil

PREPARATION In a small saucepan, bring the tea and 1 cup of water to a boil. Reduce the heat and slowly stir until the tea is thick. Strain and set aside. (You can make the tea extract in advance.) In a small bowl, combine the mayonnaise, sour cream, and oil. Stir in the thick tea.

APPLICATION Using a clean cotton ball, smooth this second coat over wrinkles and fine lines. Relax for 15 minutes, then rinse off with the milk-water mixture.

ULTIMATE SAUERKRAUT MASK

2 tablespoons sauerkraut

1 teaspoon cornstarch

PREPARATION In a small bowl, mix the ingredients together well.

APPLICATION Cover your face with this and relax for 15 minutes. Rinse off with warm water.

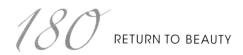

FOR WRINKLES

These recipes are specifically for women over fifty. Of course, you can enjoy them at any age! Honey and bananas are two of the best foods for combating deep lines and wrinkles.

HYDRATING HONEY MASK

1 teaspoon honey

1 teaspoon oatmeal (old-fashioned, not instant or steel-cut)

1 egg yolk

PREPARATION Mix the honey and oatmeal in a small bowl. Stir in the egg yolk and mix well.

APPLICATION Gently apply this over your face. Once the mask has dried, remove it with clean, dry cotton balls.

BANANA NO-SPLIT MASK

1 small ripe banana

2 teaspoons plain yogurt

1 teaspoon cornstarch

PREPARATION In a blender, mix together the banana, yogurt, and cornstarch.

APPLICATION Gently apply a thin layer of this over your face. Once it has dried, add a second layer, then relax for 20 to 30 minutes. Rinse off with warm water.

CURRANT-LY GORGEOUS MASK

1 teaspoon honey

2 teaspoons black currants

1 teaspoon unsalted butter

PREPARATION In a small saucepan, warm the honey over steam to liquefy it. Slowly stir in the currants. Continue stirring until the fruit is soft, then mix in the butter. Allow to cool slightly.

APPLICATION Gently apply this over your face and relax for 20 to 30 minutes. Rinse off with cold water.

HAIR CARE SOLUTIONS

The French say, "If a woman is in a bad mood, she should wash her hair!" Our hair does more than frame our beautiful faces. When we feel good about our hair, we feel good about almost everything.

Strong, shiny, beautiful hair is every woman's dream. Often, however, you can't maintain that look between visits to your hairstylist. Hormonal changes, your nervous system, and even the weather can all play a part in your hair's condition. For this reason, I've created some luxurious food rinses and hair masks that will help you maintain a happy mood!

There are three types of hair: dry, normal, and oily.

DRY HAIR tends to have split ends and grows slowly. After washing, it's not easy to style.

NORMAL HAIR has beautiful shine and elasticity. It's easy to calm and maintain in any kind of weather.

OILY HAIR is shinier than the other two types. Usually you can go only two or three days without washing it, or it looks as if you've slicked it down with oil.

DRY HAIR CARE

If you have dry hair, you should shampoo only once a week. Remember to use the masks to keep those split ends at bay!

FLOWER POWER SHAMPOO

The jasmine flower is a gentle, anti-inflammatory cleanser that calms your scalp. Honey and egg yolks are hydrating.

1 tablespoon dried jasmine

1 teaspoon honey

2 egg yolks

PREPARATION In a small saucepan, boil the dried jasmine with 1 cup of water for 5 minutes. Steep for 10 minutes and then strain. In a blender, combine the jasmine extract, honey, and egg yolks. Mix well.

APPLICATION Once a week, wash your hair with this, concentrating on your scalp. Rinse off with cold water.

CHARDONNAY RINSE

Of all the natural alcohols, white wine is the most gentle. It won't strip your hair of natural oil or treated color. Yogurt makes a creamy base for hydration with olive oil.

3 tablespoons chardonnay

1 tablespoon plain yogurt

1 teaspoon olive oil

PREPARATION In a small bowl, combine the ingredients.

APPLICATION After washing, drench your hair with this. Rinse off with cold water.

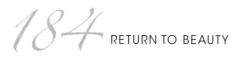

WARM COGNAC RINSE

Cognac is also a gentle natural alcohol that won't damage your hair. Warm water helps the hair absorb the egg yolk's hydration. See which rinse works better with your hair.

2 teaspoons Cognac

1 egg yolk

1 cup warm water

PREPARATION In a blender, mix the ingredients together well.

APPLICATION After shampooing, work this through your hair to the ends. Rinse off with cold water.

MS. POTATO HEAD MASK

Potatoes are packed with potassium, copper, and vitamin C. Your hair loves nutrition, too.

3 medium-sized potatoes

1 egg yolk

1 tablespoon honey

PREPARATION In a food processor or blender, puree the potatoes. Add the egg yolk and honey and mix well.

APPLICATION Pour this over your scalp, working it through to the ends, and relax for 30 minutes. Rinse off with cold water.

SATINY SMOOTH HAIR MASK

Okay, so it doesn't smell great, but your dry hair will soak up these rich oils!

1 teaspoon sesame oil

1 teaspoon fish oil

1 tablespoon sour cream

1 teaspoon baking soda

PREPARATION In a small bowl, mix together the oils, sour cream, and baking soda.

APPLICATION Massage this into your scalp, working it through to the ends, and relax for 30 minutes. Rinse off with warm water, then rinse again with cold to remove any fishy odor.

NORMAL HAIR CARE

For normal hair care, you should shampoo every two or three days. Follow with a rinse and conditioner. Use one of the masks once a week. A mask is deep-conditioning, which helps your hair maintain a healthy, luxurious shine.

ROSEMARY SHAMPOO

Rosemary is a gentle, refreshing cleanser for hair. It is even said to promote hair growth. Honey and sour cream make certain that the herb doesn't strip away any of your hair's natural oils.

2 teaspoons fresh rosemary

1 teaspoon honey

1 tablespoon sour cream

PREPARATION In a blender, combine the rosemary, honey, sour cream, and ¼ cup of water. Mix well.

APPLICATION Massage this into your hair, focusing on the scalp. Rinse off well with cold water.

HEALTHY HAIR RINSE

Apple cider vinegar stimulates hair follicles and is also great for dandruff. Mayonnaise is moisturizing and adds shine.

1 teaspoon mayonnaise

1 teaspoon apple cider vinegar

1 cup warm water

PREPARATION In a small bowl, combine the mayo, vinegar, and water. Mix well.

APPLICATION After shampooing, drench your hair with this rinse. Massage it into your scalp, working it through to the ends. Rinse off with warm water.

HONEY HAIR CONDITIONER

Honey and olive oil are great natural hair moisturizers that infuse a healthy shine. Yogurt provides a creamy conditioning base.

½ teaspoon olive oil

1 teaspoon honey

1 teaspoon plain yogurt

PREPARATION In a small bowl, mix together the oil, honey, and yogurt.

APPLICATION Apply this to your hair, making certain to focus on the ends. Rinse off with cold water.

GENTLE CHAMOMILE HAIR MASK

Chamomile infuses gentleness into everything—even hair. Hops are packed with hair vitamins, and avocado is one of the best natural moisturizers around.

1 teaspoon dried chamomile

1 teaspoon avocado, mashed

½ cup beer

PREPARATION In a small saucepan, bring the dried chamomile and 1 cup of water to a boil. Turn off the heat and steep for 10 minutes. Strain the water into a small bowl, add mashed avocado and beer, and mix well.

APPLICATION Once a week, drench your hair with this mask and relax for 20 minutes. Rinse off with cold water.

LEMONY SHINE HAIR MASK

Lemon gives your hair shine without stripping away natural oils. The egg yolk and yogurt pack a moisturizing punch.

2 tablespoons lemon juice

1 egg yolk

1 teaspoon plain yogurt

PREPARATION In a small bowl, combine the lemon juice, egg yolk, and yogurt and mix well.

APPLICATION Cover your hair with this, focusing on the ends. You can wrap your head in a towel to hold in the moisture. Relax for 20 minutes, then rinse off with warm water.

OILY HAIR CARE

To maintain a healthy look, oily hair must be washed every two or three days. These recipes contain the strongest cleansers but will not damage your hair. Experiment with the masks to see which offers the best results.

B CLEAN SHAMPOO

Egg whites work not only on oily skin but are a wonder for oily hair as well. Baking soda is a natural cleanser.

1 egg white

1 teaspoon baking soda

2 teaspoons flour

PREPARATION In a small bowl, mix the ingredients together.

APPLICATION Apply this liberally to your scalp and massage, working it through to the ends. Rinse off with cold water.

BACK TO BASIL SHAMPOO

Basil removes dirt and pollutants from your hair, leaving it feeling (and looking) rich and shiny.

½ cup warm water

1 tablespoon chopped fresh (or dried) basil

1 tablespoon honey

1 teaspoon vegetable oil

PREPARATION In a bowl, combine the warm water, basil, honey, and oil. Mix well.

APPLICATION Massage this into your scalp, working it through to the ends. Rinse off with cold water.

SHINY LIMEY SHAMPOO

Lime is a natural dandruff fighter and leaves your hair looking healthy and shiny. Warm milk is soothing.

¼ cup warm milk

1 small lime

1 egg white

1 teaspoon baking soda

PREPARATION In a food processor or blender, combine the milk, lime (with the peel), egg white, and baking soda. Blend well.

APPLICATION Cover your hair with this, working it through to the ends. Rinse off with cold water.

DILL-ICIOUS HAIR MASK

Dill has antimicrobial properties and eases tension headaches. This herb should not be used during pregnancy but is safe at all other times. This mask is like giving your hair a mini spa experience!

1 tablespoon chopped fresh (or dried) dill

1 teaspoon vodka

2 tablespoons plain yogurt

PREPARATION In a small bowl, combine the ingredients. Mix well.

APPLICATION Apply this to your scalp, making certain to focus on the ends. You may wrap your head in a towel to retain moisture if you like. Relax for 20 minutes, then rinse off with cold water.

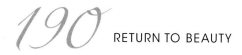

SANDWICH MASK

Wheat bread contains B vitamins, which are good for skin and hair. Dry mustard is said to be good for preventing baldness and split ends and infusing shine into dull hair. Milk soothes without making your hair oily.

2 slices wheat bread

¼ cup milk

1 teaspoon dry mustard

PREPARATION In a bowl, soak the bread in the milk. Add the mustard and ½ cup of water and mash with a fork.

APPLICATION Apply this liberally to the ends of your hair; massage any remaining mask into your scalp. Rinse off with cold water.

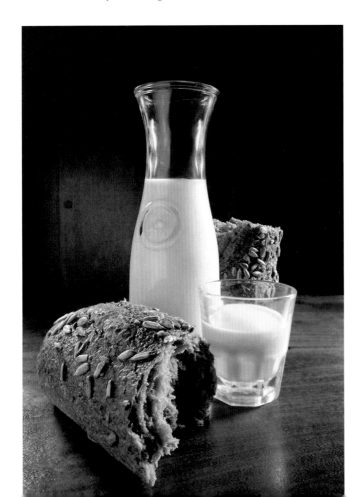

TREATED, COLORED, AND DAMAGED HAIR CARE

If your hair has lost its bounce and shine because of coloring or treatments, it's damaged. These two masks will return it to its full beauty!

REENERGIZE ME MINT HAIR RINSE

Mint refreshes and is soothing. Carrots help your hair become stronger and grow more quickly.

2 teaspoons chopped fresh (or dried) mint

1 cup warm water

1 teaspoon carrot juice

PREPARATION Add the mint to the warm water. Steep for 30 minutes, then strain. In a small bowl, combine the mint extract and carrot juice.

APPLICATION After shampooing, massage this rinse into your scalp, working it into the ends. Rinse off with warm water.

GREENS HAIR MASK

Cabbage leaves are soothing and anti-inflammatory. Spinach is packed with minerals and vitamins. Lemon juice balances your natural pH.

2 cabbage leaves

1 cup chopped spinach

½ teaspoon lemon juice

PREPARATION In a blender, combine the ingredients. Blend well.

APPLICATION Massage this into your hair, paying special attention to the ends, and relax for 1 hour. Rinse off with warm water.

HAND CARE

Of all the parts of our body, our hands often take the biggest beating. We use them to garden, cook, and clean. They are soaked in dirty dishwater, scrubbed with antibacterial soap, and left to battle the sun, cold, and wind.

For this reason, our age tends to show the most on our hands. Here are several recipes to get them looking young and supple again.

CALMING HAND SOAK

If your hands are cracked or dry, this treatment will revive them.

1 teaspoon potato starch

1 cup tepid water

2 cups boiling water

PREPARATION Mix the potato starch with the tepid water. Add the boiling water.

APPLICATION Test before soaking your hands. The water temperature should not burn your skin. Soak your hands in this for 10 to 15 minutes.

PERK-O-LATER HAND SCRUB

After enjoying your cup of morning coffee, scoop a small amount of cooled grounds into your palm. Coffee grounds are a gentle exfoliant. Rub your hands together for several minutes, then rinse off with warm water.

CREAMY ROSE HAND MASK

Rose oil is healing. Milk is soothing and comforting. Honey is a natural exfoliant. The egg yolks are for hydration.

2 teaspoons rose oil

1 teaspoon milk

1 teaspoon honey

2 egg yolks

PREPARATION In a blender, combine the ingredients. Blend until creamy.

APPLICATION Liberally cover your hands with this and relax for 10 to 15 minutes. Rinse off with warm water.

ALMONDS 'N' OATS COMFORT MASK

Oatmeal is a hydrating and soothing food. Almond oil acts as an anti-inflammatory, antiaging skin treatment.

2 teaspoons freshly cooked oatmeal

2 drops almond oil

PREPARATION In a small bowl, combine the warm oatmeal and almond oil. Allow it to cool slightly.

APPLICATION Cover your hands with this and rest for 15 minutes. Rinse off with warm water.

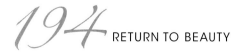

HAPPY HANDS CREAM

This treatment will leave your skin feeling flexible and supple. Butter is the ultimate moisturizer!

1 teaspoon dried chamomile

1 teaspoon unsalted butter

1 teaspoon avocado

PREPARATION In a small saucepan, bring the chamomile and 2 cups of water to a boil. Steep for 5 minutes, then strain. In a bowl, combine the chamomile extract, butter, and avocado. Mash the ingredients with a fork to mix well.

APPLICATION Apply this liberally to your hands as often as needed, especially before going to bed.

FOREVER YOUNG HAND LOTION

Coconut oil softens and gives your skin a youthful appearance. Cocoa butter is a great emollient. It smoothes wrinkles and helps thin skin remain flexible and well moisturized.

2 teaspoons coconut oil

1 teaspoon almond oil

1 teaspoon cocoa butter

PREPARATION In a small microwave-safe bowl, combine the ingredients. Heat on low power in the microwave for 2 or 3 seconds, being careful not to overheat. Stir.

APPLICATION Massage this into your hands as needed.

SPRING HANDS

If you're a gardener, try this trick every time you sink your hands into the soil.

Before gardening

Run your nails over a bar of soap and leave the soap under your nails to protect them. Put on your gloves.

After gardening

Remove the gloves. In the sink, rub a little sugar between your hands, then scrub with your soap.

YOUR HANDS HAVE NEVER LOOKED MORE BEAUTIFUL!

NAIL CARE

Strong nails come from a healthy diet. Be certain you are getting enough calcium by consuming dark leafy greens and yogurt. If your nails are thin or splitting, these treatments will help to make them resilient again.

BITTER BUTTER NAIL SOAK

Apple cider vinegar may taste bitter, but it's a proven nail builder. Butter is the best hydrator!

2 tablespoons unsalted butter

1 teaspoon apple cider vinegar

PREPARATION In a small microwave-safe bowl, melt the butter in the microwave for 1 or 2 seconds. Mix in the vinegar.

APPLICATION Test the butter to be certain it's not too hot. Soak your fingers in this for 10 minutes, then wipe off with a warm cloth.

HOT B SOAK

Baking soda is alkaline, so it neutralizes skin's acidity.

1 cup hot water

1 teaspoon baking soda

1 teaspoon apple cider vinegar

PREPARATION In a small bowl, combine the ingredients.

APPLICATION Soak your fingers in this for 15 to 20 minutes. Rinse off with warm water. Use this recipe every day for 2 weeks or until nails are restored.

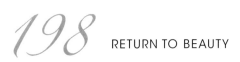

SASSY NAILS MASK

Pineapples pack a punch. High in enzymes that remove dead skin cells, they also contain vitamins A, B, and C and folic acid.

1 vitamin E capsule

1 teaspoon sour cream

1 tablespoon pineapple juice

PREPARATION Cut off the tip of the capsule and squeeze the oil into a small bowl. Stir in the sour cream and pineapple juice. Mix well.

APPLICATION Cover your nails with this and relax for 10 minutes. Rinse off with warm water.

GOOD WITCHES SCRUB

Remember that your grandmother said castor oil was good for you! It's even true for split nails. Witch hazel is a great astringent. Salt removes impurities. Honey hydrates.

1 tablespoon castor oil

1 tablespoon witch hazel

1 tablespoon salt

½ tablespoon honey

PREPARATION In a small bowl, combine the ingredients and mix well.

APPLICATION Rub this into your nail and cuticle area for 5 to 10 minutes. Do not rinse off. Wipe off with a clean cloth.

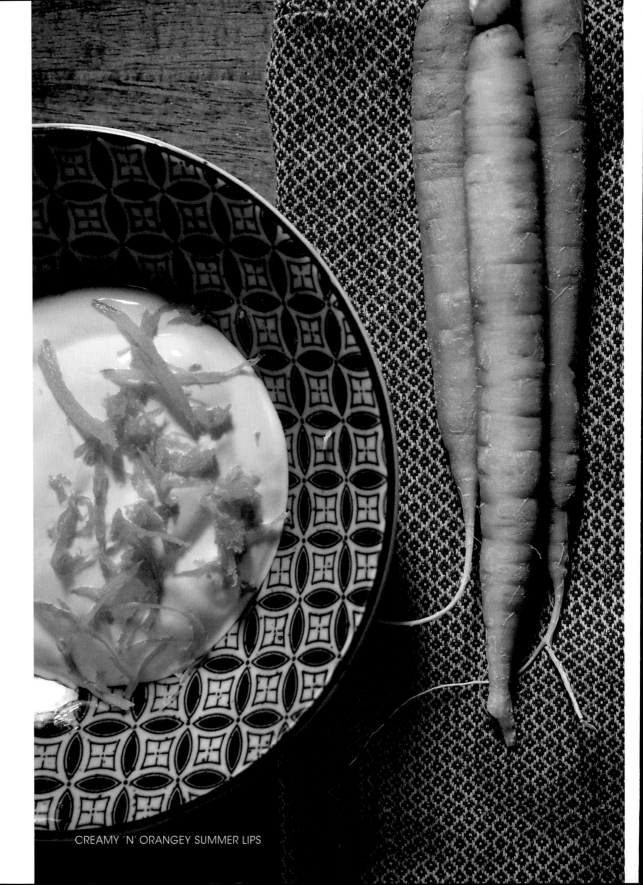

CREAMY 'N' ORANGEY SUMMER LIPS

LIP CARE

Shiny, plump, healthy lips—these days woman will do (and pay) almost anything to achieve great-looking lips. Here's the secret.

Having naturally beautiful lips isn't that hard. You must remember to take good care of them. Sun, wind, pollution, and dirt cause thin lines to form, which eventually become deep wrinkles—especially as you grow older. Just like the rest of your face, the skin on your lips requires soothing protection from the elements. Make certain that your lipstick contains sunscreen.

Regular care combined with using the right products will help your lips keep their beautiful natural shape and shine.

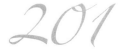

LIP HYDRATION MASKS

Once lips start to crack or peel, even the most expensive lipsticks will not help them rehydrate. These three masks offer special healing and moisturizing remedies. Choose the one you need based upon your lips' condition. Apply once a week and continue until you're smiling again.

JUST JUICY RED

The lactic acid in dairy hydrates and exfoliates simultaneously, while beet juice infuses your lips with vitamins A and C.

½ teaspoon cottage cheese

½ teaspoon sour cream

½ teaspoon beet juice

Rose oil

PREPARATION In a small bowl, combine the cottage cheese, sour cream, and beet juice. Mix well.

APPLICATION Pat over the lip area with your fingertips. Relax for 15 minutes. Rinse with warm water. Smooth a few drops of rose oil over your lips to seal in the moisture.

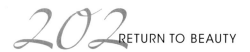

HEALING HONEY WINTER HYDRATOR

The anti-inflammatory properties of cucumber and honey soothe chapped lips back to supple again.

1 teaspoon shredded cucumber

½ teaspoon honey

½ teaspoon sour cream

Almond oil

PREPARATION In a small bowl, combine the cucumber, honey, and sour cream. Mix well.

APPLICATION Pat over the lip area with your fingertips. Relax for 15 minutes. Rinse with warm water. Smooth a few drops of almond oil over your lips to seal in the moisture.

CREAMY 'N' ORANGEY SUMMER LIPS

Whether you're a gardener or a sun goddess, the beta-carotene in carrots provides antioxidant properties, and Greek yogurt moisturizes and exfoliates.

1 teaspoon shredded carrot

½ teaspoon Greek yogurt

Lavender oil

PREPARATION In a small bowl, combine the carrot and yogurt. Mix well.

APPLICATION Pat over the lip area with your fingertips. Relax for 15 minutes. Rinse with warm water. Smooth a few drops of lavender oil over your lips to seal in the moisture.

LIP FIXES

SMOOTH ME

Once a week, pat honey over your lip area. Take a small, gentle lip brush and scrub away the peeling or dry skin. Now try the quick rinse.

QUICK RINSE

Combine ½ teaspoon of cucumber juice and ½ teaspoon of carrot juice. Add ½ teaspoon of sour cream. Dab over your lips. Leave on for 10 minutes, then rinse off with cool water. Pat olive oil over your lips.

SASSY SHINE

There are plenty of glosses on the market created to make your lips shine. Most of them are also very sticky. This is a real problem for women with long hair—every time you turn your head you have to pull your hair away from your sticky lips! There is a simple remedy: In your palm, mix a little softened butter with some rose oil. Smooth it over your lip area. Beautiful!

KISS ME GLOSS

Here's a sweet, sexy recipe for great-looking lips.

1 vitamin E capsule

1 teaspoon cocoa butter

¼ teaspoon grated chocolate

PREPARATION Cut off the tip of the capsule. Squeeze the oil from the capsule into a small microwave-safe bowl, then add the cocoa butter and chocolate. Microwave for only a few seconds to melt. Test for temperature.

APPLICATION Smooth this over your lip area—now you're ready to be kissed!

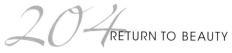

HEALTHY HAPPY FEET FIXES

Our feet carry us through our lives. It's so important to take good care of them. Many women pay for pedicures to keep their feet looking nice, but in order to maintain optimum health, feet need extra tender loving care, especially in colder weather.

HAPPY HEELS

This little mask will make you click your heels!

Simply shred 1 ripe tomato and spread it over your heel area, especially over the cracked or peeling areas. Wrap your feet in clean gauze and prop them up for 30 minutes. Rinse with tepid water (never put hot water on dry feet!). Pat dry with a soft cloth, then apply your cream.

HAPPY HEELS TWO

One or two times a week, wash your feet with this recipe.

Mix 2 tablespoons of vodka with 1 teaspoon of baking soda. Cover your heels with this, wrap them in clean gauze, and relax for 30 minutes. Rinse off with tepid water. Pat dry with a soft cloth, then apply your cream.

TOES TOO!

Our little digits can get painful cracks if we're not careful. Here's a wonderful toe mask that will keep them soft and pink. This is the perfect remedy to try before bedtime.

Take 1 cup of milk and 1 small apple. Slice the apple and cook it in the milk on the stove until it softens. Drain. Mash the apple and add 1 teaspoon of corn oil. Massage this over your toes, then cover them in clean gauze or a small towel and rest for 30 minutes. Rinse with tepid water, then apply your cream.

BUMPS AWAY

Some people suffer from bunions or develop little bumps on their feet. The garlic in this recipe will frighten them all away!

Soak your feet in hot water for 15 minutes (be careful not to burn yourself). Shred 1 onion and put 1 garlic clove through a garlic press. In a small bowl, mash the ingredients together. Cover the trouble spots with this and relax for 15 minutes. Rinse off and use a pumice stone, then soften your feet with olive oil. Put on socks and go to sleep.

MASHED POTATO FOOT MASK

This mask can be used once a week to keep your feet soft and healthy.

Cube an unpeeled potato and boil in 1 cup of water for 15 minutes. Drain. Mash the potato, adding 1 teaspoon of sea salt and 1 teaspoon of milk. Cover your feet with the mashed potato mixture, then cover with clean gauze and prop them up for 20 minutes. Rinse off with tepid water, then apply your cream.

"MOSES SUPPOSES HIS TOESES ARE ROSES"

Women want to have lovely feet, but sometimes after a long day in leather shoes, our toes smell a little less than rosy! Here's a simple rinse that helps them maintain a sweet aroma! Use right before bedtime.

In a blender, combine a quartered lemon, ½ cup of milk, ½ teaspoon of cinnamon, and 1 tablespoon of corn oil. Rinse your feet with this. Don't rinse off with water.

PAIN AWAY

After standing all day in heels, or walking or jogging around the park, our feet hurt! Chop 2 cabbage leaves, place them in a small bowl, and add 1 tablespoon of warm vegetable oil. Wrap the mixture in clean gauze, place on the painful area, and rest for 30 minutes. This remedy takes the pain away.

EXTRA TIRED LEGS

I would be remiss if I didn't include a recipe for those days when it isn't just your feet that hurt—your legs are also tired.

Take 2 large bowls. Fill each with hot water, 1 tablespoon dried chamomile, and 1 teaspoon of sea salt. Soak your feet for 15 minutes. Then fill 2 bowls with cold water. Soak your feet for 15 minutes. You can do this up to ten times, or until the ache in your legs subsides.

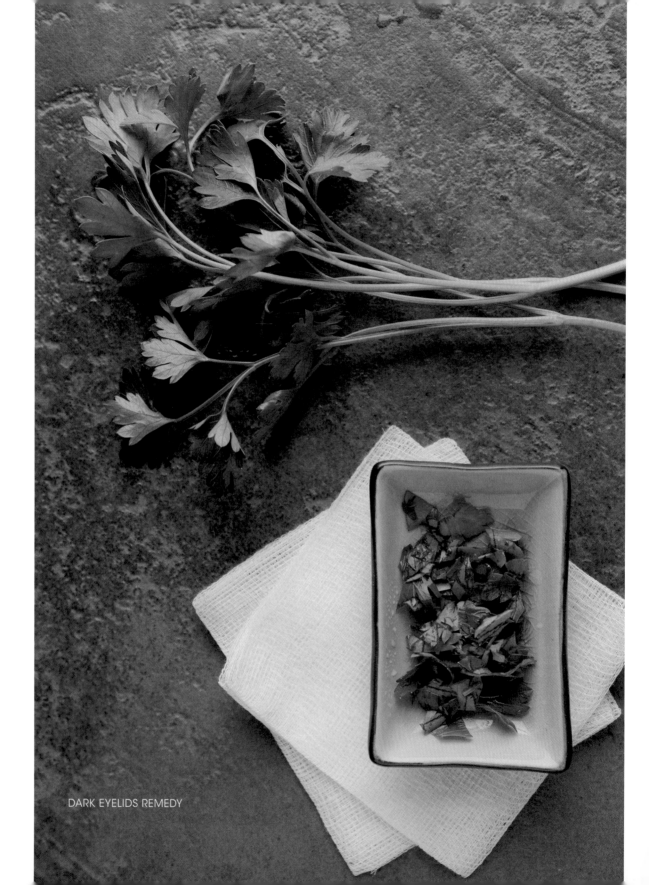

DARK EYELIDS REMEDY

EYE CARE

If we are fortunate enough to have our eyesight, we are able to enjoy all of the world's magnificence and beauty. My son's smile, the canyons I drive through after work, even my husband snoring on the sofa—I take in my life with my own beautiful eyes.

Happy, sad, worried, or frightened—these windows to the soul also tell others all they need to know about us. If your eyes are watery, this means there are vitamins missing from your diet. Also, the older we get, the drier our eyes can become. These problems can be fixed with adjustments in our lifestyle and diet.

We need to take good care of our eyes. Good eye vitamins are A, E, C, B, and B_2. Foods that are rich in these vitamins include carrots, green beans, green onions, melons, tomatoes, bananas, potatoes, cabbage, wheat, walnuts, garlic, chicken, pinto beans, milk, and fish.

Avoiding the following habits will help your eyes maintain health: overworking, too much computer time, too much television time, smoking, alcohol, and not enough sleep.

EYE REMEDIES

TIRED EYES

To rejuvenate your eyes after a long day, fill a large bowl with water and add 1 teaspoon of sea salt. Soak your face in the water, opening and closing your eyes several times. Soak clean cotton balls in green tea and swipe them over closed eyes.

PUMPKIN EYE MASK

Peel and seed a slice of pumpkin. Cook it in 2 cups of water until soft, then mash it and add 1 teaspoon of honey. Place inside clean gauze, then place over your eyes and relax for 20 minutes.

POTATO EYE MASK

Peel 1 small potato. Shred it, then place it in clean gauze. Cover your eyes with this and relax for 15 minutes. Rinse off with cold chamomile tea.

RED IRRITATED EYES

In a small bowl, mix 1 teaspoon of chopped parsley and 1 cup of milk. Soak clean cotton balls in the mixture and swipe them over closed eyes.

REMEDIES FOR DARK CIRCLES

As well as changing those habits that help to create dark pigmentation under the eyes, try one or all of these recipes. (Sometimes darkness under our eyes or on our eyelids is genetic, but these recipes help lighten its appearance.)

DARK EYELIDS

Place 2 teaspoons of chopped fresh parsley on your eyelids and rest for 20 to 25 minutes. Rinse off with warm water.

DARK UNDER-EYE CIRCLES

Place 2 teaspoons of organic cottage cheese on clean cotton balls. Pat gently under your eyes and leave on for 20 minutes. Rinse off with warm water.

OR

In a small saucepan, put 3 teaspoons of diced cucumber into 1 cup of water. Bring to a boil, then simmer for 15 minutes. Mix in 1 teaspoon of honey. Allow to cool. Dip a cotton ball in the mixture and pat gently under your eye area. Leave on for 5 to 10 minutes. Rinse off with cold water.

LASHES AND BROWS

We have to remember to take care of all the parts of our faces—even our lashes and brows.

Our lashes protect our eyes. To maintain healthy, thick lashes, it's important that you wash off your eye makeup before bed every night.

After washing off your eye makeup, put a little castor oil on your fingertip and massage it into your eyebrows. Smooth a little over your lashes, too. Or you can try camphor oil instead.

For shiny brows and lashes, dip a clean cotton ball in warm almond or peach oil. Pat over your brows and lashes and relax for 10 to 15 minutes. Rinse off with warm water.

Sleep tight!

NECK CARE

More than our faces, our necks reveal our age. As we get older, our skin loses its elasticity and fine lines begin to appear—especially if our skin is dry.

Before we move on to the recipes, I want to give you some of my grandmother's rules for keeping your neck graceful and smooth well into old age.

First rule—never read a book lying down. This presses your neck into your chest, shortening the muscles and elongating them in the back. Don't stop reading great literature and learning new things—just read sitting up. Purchase an inexpensive book table.

Second rule—walk like an Egyptian. In ancient Egypt and Africa, women were renowned for their graceful, long necks. How did they achieve them? They carried everything on their heads! Place a book on your head and walk around the house. It may seem silly, but you'll be training your neck muscles and creating great posture at the same time.

Third rule—hot and cold compresses do help. Place a washcloth in hot water, then wrap it around your neck. Relax until it cools. Repeat using cold water.

GRACEFUL NECK REGIMEN

PERFECTLY GREEN MASK

1 teaspoon chopped parsley

1 cup warm milk

PREPARATION In a small bowl, mix the ingredients together.

APPLICATION Dip a washcloth in the mixture, then pat over your neck area. Leave on until dry. Rinse off with warm water, then apply the Graceful Swan Cream (opposite).

EGG AND POTATOES MASK

2 baked potatoes, skin on

1 egg yolk

1 teaspoon olive oil

1 teaspoon honey

PREPARATION In a bowl, mash the baked potatoes. Mix in the egg yolk, oil, and honey. Mash together well.

APPLICATION Apply this liberally over your neck area. Cover with plastic wrap to retain moisture, and relax for 15 to 20 minutes. Rinse off with warm water, then apply the Graceful Swan Cream (opposite).

GRACEFUL SWAN CREAM

1 teaspoon dried chamomile

1 teaspoon cocoa butter

1 teaspoon honey

1 teaspoon olive oil

½ teaspoon witch hazel

PREPARATION In a small saucepan, bring the dried chamomile and ½ cup of water to a boil. Steep for 10 minutes, then strain. In a small microwave-safe bowl, melt the cocoa butter in the microwave to soften. Add the honey, oil, and witch hazel. Add the chamomile extract and mix well.

APPLICATION Gently apply this over your neck area after cleansing and before bed every night.

CUCUMBER WASH AND TONE

1 large cucumber

3 teaspoons vodka

PREPARATION Shred the cucumber with the skin on. In a clean container, mix the ingredients together. Leave in a cool, dark place for 10 days, then refrigerate.

APPLICATION Smooth this over your neck using clean cotton balls. Do not rinse off.

CREAMY YOLK WASH

1 teaspoon sour cream

1 egg yolk

1 teaspoon lemon juice

PREPARATION In a small bowl, mix the sour cream and egg yolk together, then add the lemon juice. Mix well.

APPLICATION Wash your neck with this, then rinse off with cold water.

 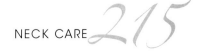

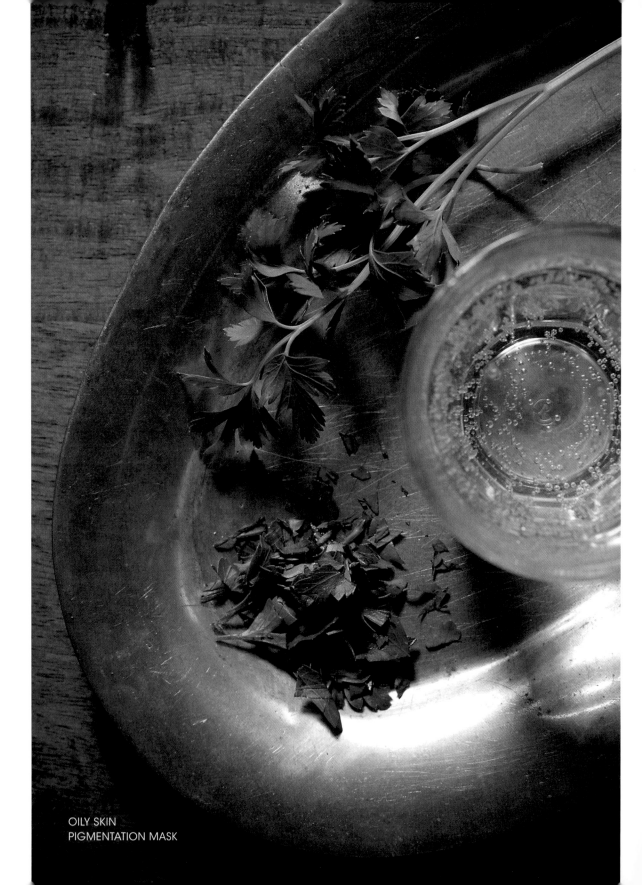

OILY SKIN
PIGMENTATION MASK

FRECKLES AND DARK SPOTS

If you love your freckles (they are unique and beautiful!) but wish they were a little lighter, the recipes below are for you.

As we age we often begin to notice dark spots (some people call them age spots) on our skin. These can be due to hormonal changes or too much time spent in the sun during youth.

Whether they are freckles or dark spots, these two remedies lighten pigmentation:

1. Squeeze a fresh grapefruit. Every morning and evening, dip a clean cotton ball in the juice and smooth it over your face.
2. Cut 1 slice of honeydew melon and mash it in a small bowl. Place this inside clean gauze and leave on the area for 20 minutes.

ANGEL KISSES MASK

1 slice whole wheat bread

¼ cup milk

PREPARATION Soak the bread slice in the milk for 1 hour, then mash it with your hands.

APPLICATION Cover the area and relax for 20 minutes. Rinse off with cold water.

SHARP C TONER

1 tablespoon wine vinegar

4 tablespoons water

2 tablespoons lemon juice

PREPARATION In a small bowl, mix the ingredients together.

APPLICATION Gently smooth this over the area, using a clean cotton ball, every morning and evening.

CLEAR C TONER

1 cucumber

1 onion

PREPARATION In a blender or food processor, puree the cucumber, then pour the juice into a small container. Puree the onion and pour the juice into another small container. Combine 1 tablespoon of each. You may refrigerate the remaining juices to use for a week.

APPLICATION Gently smooth this over the area, using a clean cotton ball, every morning and evening.

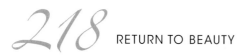

OILY SKIN PIGMENTATION MASK

1 tablespoon chopped parsley

1 tablespoon honey

PREPARATION In a small bowl, mix the ingredients together.

APPLICATION Apply this to the affected areas and leave it on for 20 minutes. Rinse off with cold water.

DRY SKIN PIGMENTATION MASK

1 tablespoon chopped parsley

1 tablespoon sour cream

PREPARATION In a small bowl, mix the ingredients together.

APPLICATION Apply this to the affected areas and leave it on for 20 minutes. Rinse off with cold water.

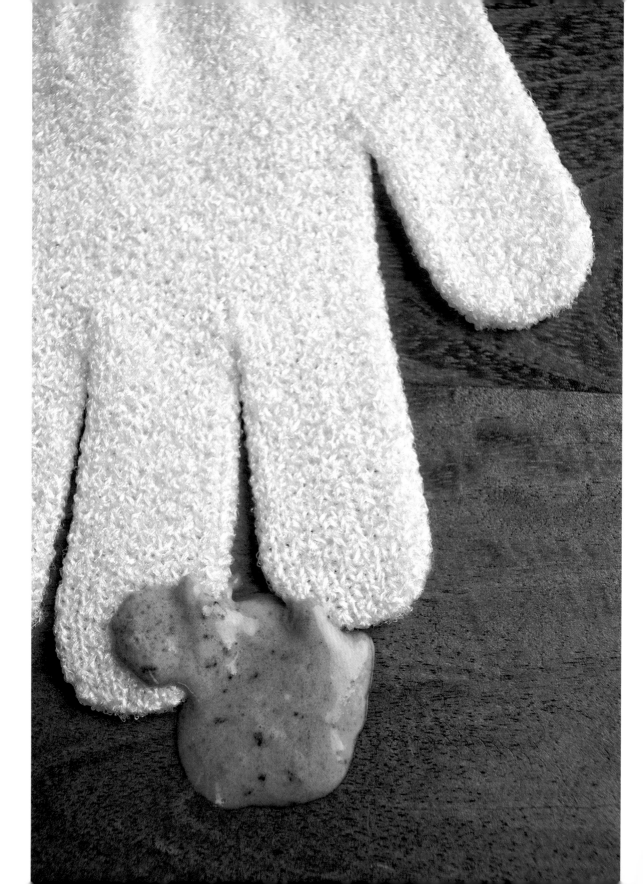

QUICK FACE TAN

Looking a little gray after working indoors all week? Have a hot date? Feeling blue? Add a sunburst of health and beauty to your face with this quick mask.

SUMMER GLOW MASK

Pour fresh-squeezed carrot juice into a bowl. Take a large piece of clean gauze and cut out holes for your eyes and mouth. Soak the gauze in the carrot juice and wring out any excess liquid. Lay it gently over your face for 10 minutes. Repeat the process until your skin is the desired color. This routine should be done every day, using a clean piece of gauze each time, for continued results.

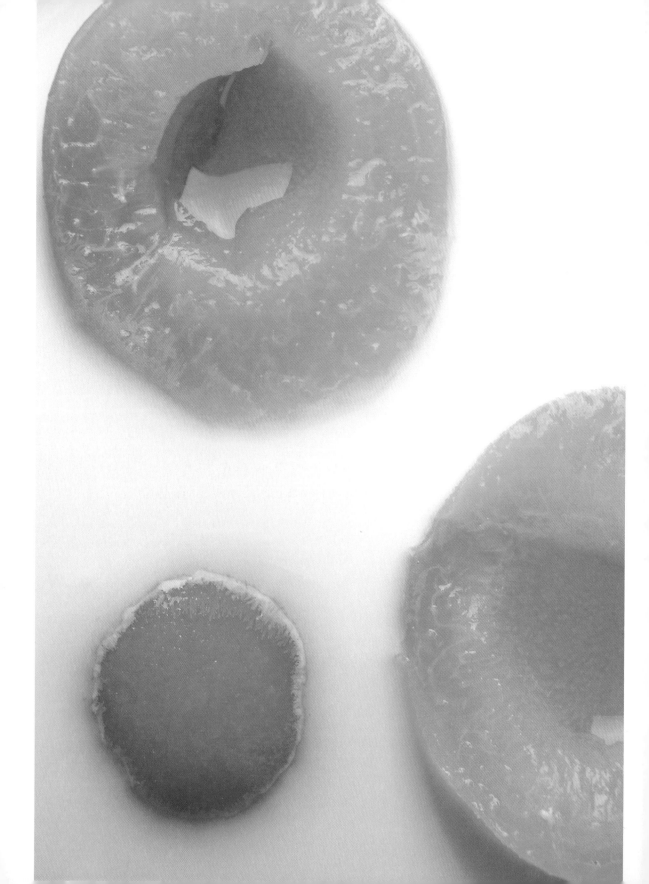

Part 4

PREGNANCY

New life is growing inside your body. This miraculous event brings about hormonal changes that affect your hair, nails, and skin. When I was pregnant with my son, I learned which foods were the most important for both of us. Everything I put in, and on, my body went into his little body as well, so I was not going to use any products that contained artificial ingredients! We all want our babies to be born healthy and grow up happy. Good self-care is the first nurturing you give to your unborn child. For this reason, I wanted to include a section for mothers-to-be. By following these simple recipes, you can minimize everything from skin discolorations to varicose veins, and even stretch marks. For changes in your hair and nails, you can turn to the Simple Solutions section (page 171).

Taking good care of your health during this time allows you to really enjoy the process. Think good thoughts. Dwell on happy things. Remember to be grateful.

Relax! In nine months, the real work begins!

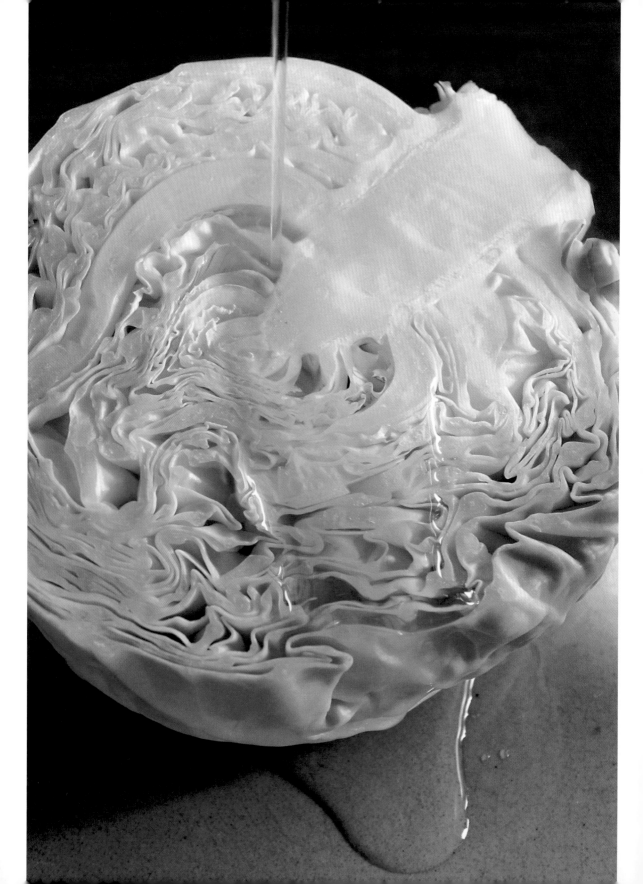

PREGNANCY SELF-CARE

Whatever is happening inside our bodies eventually shows up on our faces. For women who are pregnant, this is even more pronounced. If you have oily skin, it gets oilier, developing pimples and blackheads. If you have dry skin, you begin to find flaky patches everywhere. Don't worry—there are easy remedies for these concerns. First, let's cover the basics.

EAT WELL

During this time you need vitamins, especially A and C. Vitamin A can be found in many fresh foods, including fish oil, butter, egg yolks, carrots, green onions, spinach, lettuce, and apricots. A high concentration of vitamin C can be found in cabbage, green onions, spinach, tomatoes, strawberries, raspberries, tangerines, oranges, lemons, apples, and red meat.

Also, make certain to eat plenty of yogurt.

TAKE WALKS

It's important to take walks in the fresh air, even though you must remember to protect your skin from the harmful effects of the sun. You need the sun's vitamin D right now.

WATCH HAPPY MOVIES

Also read funny books and listen to lighthearted music that keeps your toes tapping.

BASIC SKIN CARE REGIMEN

Keep your skin clean and hydrated

1. When you wake up in the morning, first wash your upper body with a soft washcloth. Use only warm water, no soap. This is especially important in your last trimester.
2. When you're ready, please shower. It's best during pregnancy not to take hot baths or sit in a hot tub. Use a mild, chemical-free soap. Moisturize with the recipes on page 228.
3. Once a week, use a loofah in the shower to remove dead skin cells.
4. Each night before going to bed, rinse your hands, feet, and neck with warm water. Choose one of the pregnancy toners (pages 231, 232, and 234) and use it every night as well.
5. If you were already prone to skin troubles, during your pregnancy they can sometimes get worse. Because of the extra hormones, pregnant women need to be vigilant about keeping the face clean, washing every morning and evening.

BABY MAMA'S BEAUTIFUL FACE CREAM

Before you leave the house each day, remember to use this hydrating, gentle cream to protect your dry skin.

1 tablespoon Greek yogurt

1 teaspoon lemon juice

1 teaspoon rose oil

PREPARATION In a small bowl, combine the ingredients and mix well.

APPLICATION Apply this gently over your face and neck after showering.

BABY MAMA'S BEAUTIFUL BODY CREAM

When you're pregnant, it might seem as if all of the moisture has left your body! This lotion will infuse hydration and healthiness into your dry skin, keeping it soft and supple.

2 small cucumbers

2 teaspoons olive oil

1 egg yolk

1 teaspoon flour

PREPARATION Peel and chop the cucumbers. In a blender, combine the cucumbers, oil, egg yolk, and flour. Mix well.

APPLICATION After showering, apply this cream generously all over your body.

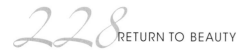

For pimples or breakouts, use this mask once a week:

REMBRANDT'S ROSE MASK

A pregnant mother's face is more beautiful than the greatest of paintings. This mask will even your skin tone, tighten and close the pores, and leave you feeling soft.

2 teaspoons dried rose petals

1 onion slice

1 teaspoon honey

1 egg white

½ cup warm water

1 teaspoon flour

PREPARATION In a blender, combine the petals, onion, honey, egg white, and water. Slowly stir in the flour to make a thick paste.

APPLICATION Cover your face and neck with this and relax for 20 minutes. Rinse off with warm water.

GLOW

People smile when you pass. There are roses in your cheeks. The hormonal imbalance has caused your oil glands to produce more oil, which creates that beautiful pregnancy "glow." To maintain your skin's pH balance, use this mask when needed.

BALANCING MASK

Honey is great for older skin, but it's also a nice exfoliant. Sour cream lightens skin tone and is hydrating.

1 teaspoon honey

1 teaspoon sour cream

PREPARATION In a small bowl, blend the ingredients together well.

APPLICATION Gently apply this to your face and relax for 20 minutes. Rinse off with warm water.

Dry Skin and Normal-to-Dry Skin Toners

If you have dry skin, you really love the glow! For the first time in your life, all you have to do is keep it simple.

GORGEOUS GLOW TONER

Health-infusing parsley with a dash of natural alcohol is the best toner for pregnant women with dry or normal-to-dry skin.

2 tablespoons chopped parsley

½ cup mineral water

2 teaspoons vodka

PREPARATION In a small bowl, mix the parsley with the vodka, then add the mineral water.

APPLICATION Before bedtime, apply this to your face using a clean cotton ball.

ORANGE YOU HAPPY TONER

If you prefer oranges to parsley, or want to mix it up a bit, here's another wonderful toner to add to your regimen. Vitamin C is mandatory for women who are expecting.

1 ripe orange

¼ cup vodka

½ cup water

PREPARATION In a blender or food processor, puree the orange, peel and all. Transfer the mixture to a small bowl and add the vodka. Store in a dark cupboard, in a clean glass container, for 5 to 7 days. Add the water.

APPLICATION Every night before bed, wipe this over your face using a clean cotton ball.

Oily Skin and Normal-to-Oily Skin Toner

If your skin is oily, that glow can light up the night! First, you have to cut down on fried foods and sweets, especially chocolate. The third trimester can be particularly difficult for mothers-to-be with oily skin. It's very important for you to remember to get plenty of B vitamins in addition to C.

TART 'N' LOVELY TONER

Apple cider vinegar helps maintain your skin's optimal pH balance. The tightening effects of natural alcohol combined with citric acid will close pores and make your breakouts disappear.

¼ cup vodka

1 tablespoon apple cider vinegar

1 tablespoon lemon juice

PREPARATION In a clean plastic bottle, combine the ingredients and shake well.

APPLICATION Twice a day, wipe your face with this using a clean cotton ball. Continue as long as needed.

STRETCH MARKS

As the baby grows and you gain the necessary weight, your skin begins to stretch. These marks are the most common skin change during pregnancy. Stretch marks appear on every woman's body in different places. Some women get them on the thighs and buttocks, others on the stomach. There are several recipes you can use to minimize their appearance.

COCOA-E BUTTER LOTION

Cocoa butter is sensual and hydrating. When combined with the healing effects of vitamin E, it can prevent stretch marks from appearing.

3 vitamin E capsules

2 tablespoons cocoa butter

PREPARATION Cut off the ends of the capsules and squeeze the oil into a small bowl. Add the cocoa butter and stir well.

APPLICATION Cover your thighs, hips, and stomach area with this every night before bed.

FLAWLESS OIL

The high vitamin E content in apricot kernel oil helps your skin maintain elasticity and clarity and, along with sesame oil, stay soft and supple. Both oils can also be used later—on baby!

1 teaspoon sesame oil

1 teaspoon apricot kernel oil

½ teaspoon honey

PREPARATION In a small bowl, combine the ingredients and mix well.

APPLICATION Apply this generously over your stretch marks to diffuse their appearance.

PIGMENTATION

Changes in the pigmentation of your skin can happen anytime during the nine months, but they are most obvious when your second trimester falls in the springtime.

A lack of vitamin C can be one reason for those skin spots during pregnancy. In order to restore balance, be certain to eat foods like cabbage, green onions, spinach, tomatoes, strawberries, raspberries, tangerines, oranges, lemons, apples, and red meat.

BERRY LIGHT MASK

Berries infuse vitamin C into your bloodstream. Honey is a sweet exfoliant.

1 tablespoon raspberries

1 tablespoon strawberries

1 teaspoon honey

PREPARATION In a blender, combine the ingredients and mix well.

APPLICATION Apply this gently over your face and neck and relax for 20 minutes. Rinse off with warm water. Use weekly if needed.

FROSTY WHITE TONER

If the smell bothers you, you don't have to use this toner. However, onion juice is the best food you can use to lighten dark patches.

1 small white onion

¼ cup witch hazel

PREPARATION In a food processor, puree the onion. Strain the juice into a clean plastic container, add the witch hazel, and refrigerate.

APPLICATION Wipe your face several times a day with this, using a clean cotton ball. Wait 10 minutes, then rinse off with warm water. Continue as long as needed.

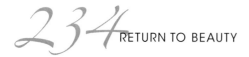

CARROT SALAD MASK

Carrots contain beta-carotene. They also offer protection from the sun. Lemon juice is an excellent source of vitamin C and offers natural bleaching.

1 small carrot

1 tablespoon lemon juice

PREPARATION Shred the carrot. In a small bowl, mix the carrot with the lemon juice.

APPLICATION Cover your face and neck with this and relax for 20 minutes. Rinse off with warm water, then apply your moisturizer.

WHITE RICE WASH

White rice acts as natural bleach on skin. This is a safe wash to use for pigmentation when you're pregnant.

2 teaspoons white rice

PREPARATION Soak the rice in 2 cups of water in a bowl overnight.

APPLICATION Wash your face with this every morning, then rinse off with warm water.

TUMMY TREATMENT

As your baby grows, your belly grows as well. Your skin stretches and gets tight, causing your abdomen to feel uncomfortable and itchy. Keep your tummy moisturized by following the steps of this natural anti-itch treatment.

CALM MY TUMMY WASH

Milk is soothing. When combined with oats, it diffuses skin irritations.

1 cup milk

2 tablespoons oatmeal (old-fashioned, not instant or steel-cut)

PREPARATION In a small microwave-safe bowl, warm the milk and ½ cup of water in the microwave. Allow to cool slightly. Add the oatmeal to the tepid milk.

APPLICATION Wash this over your abdomen using a soft washcloth.

TUMMY TAMER MASK

Cucumbers are calming. Potatoes are packed with vitamin C, which is a natural anti-inflammatory. Salt is a gentle scrub.

2 small cucumbers

1 potato

2 teaspoons salt

PREPARATION Peel the cucumbers and potato, then shred both into a bowl. Add the salt and mix well.

APPLICATION Pat this over your abdominal area and relax for 15 minutes. Wash off with warm water.

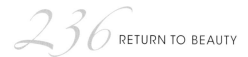

NIGHTY-NIGHT TUMMY MOISTURIZER

Lavender makes us feel serene. It is great for healing and softening skin.

2 tablespoons dried lavender

½ cup plain yogurt

1 teaspoon olive oil

PREPARATION In a small saucepan, bring the dried lavender and 1 cup of water to a boil. Steep for 10 minutes, then strain and cool. Add the yogurt and oil to the lavender water.

APPLICATION Pat this over your abdominal area every night before bed.

VARICOSE VEINS

Yes, you're gaining weight, just like the baby needs you to—but you could really do without those dark veins in your legs! Varicose veins usually show up during the second trimester. Here are a few tips to reduce their appearance.

1. Whenever you sit down to rest, elevate your legs.
2. Wear support stockings.
3. Take a walk in the fresh air before going to bed.
4. Try to avoid overeating, especially fattening foods. You want to gain a healthy amount of weight during your pregnancy. This is different from using pregnancy as an excuse to get very heavy. Heaviness increases the chance that you will get varicose veins, and makes it harder to lose them after the baby is born.
5. Eat tomatoes, which are good for blood circulation. You can drink tomato juice every day.
6. Cook 1 cup of barley in 2 cups of water. Allow it to cool and then mash it up. Apply the mixture to your legs, cover with clean gauze, and rest for 20 minutes. Rinse off with warm water.

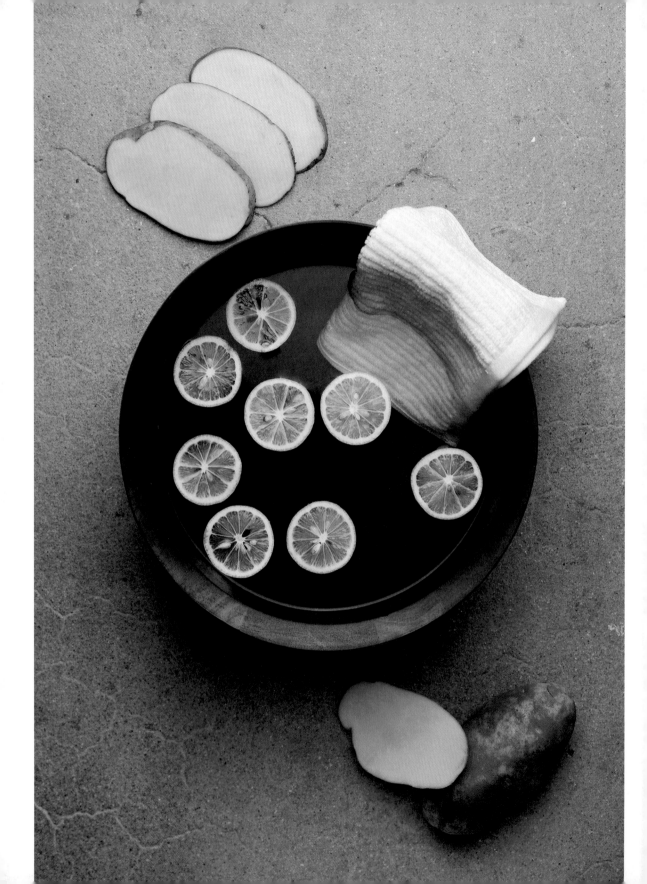

Part 5
HOW TO GIVE
YOURSELF A FACIAL

Old-world skin care traditions have always included time for rest and rejuvenation—not as a luxury but as a necessity. The pace of today's world makes it almost impossible for women to take the time to get the necessary nutrition and pampering required to stay glowing with youthful vitality. Giving yourself a facial is a gift that will make you feel, and look, wonderful on many levels.

This facial is for the times when you either can't afford a professional facial or simply don't have a reasonable hour open for an appointment at the local spa. I've created it especially for you from my twenty years of experience helping people feel beautiful. It's easy and contains a few of my little secrets.

Before you begin, choose a good location—either the bathroom or the kitchen. Remember, if you choose the bathroom, you will have to make your products in the kitchen and carry them in with you.

FACIAL PREPARATION 10 EASY STEPS

1. From either the Seasons section or the Sun Signs section, make your cleanser, moisturizer, and scrub recipes.

2. Shred 1 cucumber into a bowl. This will be used for your eyes.

3. For an oily skin peel: Shred 1 tomato, add 1 teaspoon of apple cider vinegar, and wrap the mixture in a clean piece of gauze.

4. For a dry skin peel: Peel and pit a papaya, then cube. Add a little olive oil, and wrap the mixture in a clean piece of gauze.

5. In a small bowl, combine 2 tablespoons of plain yogurt with 1 teaspoon of olive oil.

6. In another small bowl, combine 1 teaspoon of sour cream with 1 teaspoon of honey for a mask.

7. Get a clean washcloth and a clean face towel.

8. Pull your hair back into a ponytail or tuck it into a shower cap. You can even make a hair mask to wear, if you'd like, while you do your facial.

9. Wear a soft warm robe or a comfortable housedress.

10. Unless you have a ministeamer, I'm not going to ask you to put your face in hot steam at home. Please have dried lavender, chamomile, or eucalyptus oil with you.

Now, turn the page to begin your facial.

FACIAL 10 EASY STEPS

1. Wash your face with your cleanser recipe, then rinse off with warm water. Remove your eye makeup with any kind of oil and clean cotton pads.

2. Fill your sink with hot tap water. Add lavender, chamomile, or eucalyptus oil. Soak the face towel in the water and cover your face for 1 minute. Soak the towel and reapply two more times.

3. Now it's time to exfoliate with your homemade scrub. Using your fingers, move in a circular motion over your face, concentrating on the areas around your chin, nose, and forehead. If you have dry skin, be very gentle. You should scrub for 5 minutes to get the pores cleaned, then wash your face with warm water and a washcloth or a new towel.

4. Remove the tomato or papaya from the gauze. Cover your face with the tomato (oily skin peel) or the papaya (dry skin peel). Now cover your face with the gauze and rest for 10 minutes. Rinse off with warm water.

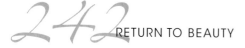

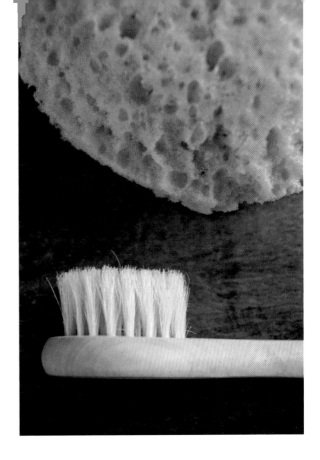

5. Now it's time to soothe your skin. Massage the plain yogurt–olive oil mixture over your face for 5 minutes. Remove with a dry soft tissue or a dry cloth.

6. Gently cover your face with the sour cream and honey mask.

7. Wrap the shredded cucumber in clean gauze (like a burrito) and place it over your eyes.

8. Relax for 20 to 25 minutes.

9. Remove the eye mask, then rinse the mask from your face with warm water. Apply your moisturizer.

10. Look at yourself in the mirror and repeat, "I am so beautiful!"

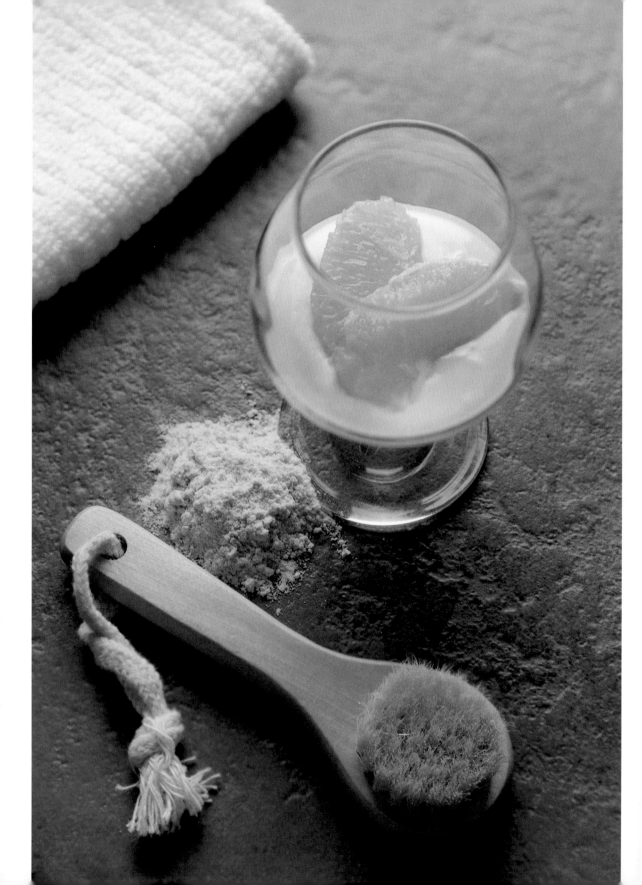

Part 6

NO FRILLS FOR MEN

It's supposed to be a secret, but I know something that men rarely share with others: They want to feel good about how they look, too.

Over the years, I have given many facials to men, usually as a birthday present or treat from a partner or friend. They have always returned for more treatments. When you're eating well, getting enough rest, and using healthy skin care products, you feel more self-confident. Even if a man is shy, when he feels good about himself, it registers with others. There is nothing sexier than a man brimming with confidence!

This section offers some quick, easy, no-frills recipes just for you. Be careful—you might get addicted. If you do, feel free to try any of the recipes in this book (maybe not those in the pregnancy section). Experiment with what works best for you.

You are lucky—your skin doesn't require that much care for it to look youthful and healthy.

SKIN CARE OILY SKIN

It's simple. Keep it clean. Follow the regimen below. Don't forget to scrub.

SIMPLY CLEAN

1 tablespoon nonfat plain yogurt

1 teaspoon lemon juice

PREPARATION In a small bowl, mix the ingredients together.

APPLICATION Pour a small amount of this onto a clean wet washcloth or sponge. Gently wash your face, then rinse with cold water.

GIN AND TONIC TONER

2 tablespoons gin

¼ cup tonic water

PREPARATION In a small bowl, mix the ingredients together.

APPLICATION Dip a clean cotton ball in the toner, then wipe it over your face. Do not rinse off.

MORNIN' DARLIN' SCRUB

1 teaspoon coffee grounds

1 teaspoon sour cream

1 teaspoon honey

PREPARATION After you've poured yourself a cup, dump the grounds into a small bowl to cool. In another small bowl, mix the sour cream and honey together, then stir in the grounds.

APPLICATION Scoop the mixture into your palms and scrub your face with it using your fingers. Rinse off with cold water.

CLEAR SKIN MASK

1 egg white

1 teaspoon lemon juice

PREPARATION In a small bowl, mix the ingredients together.

APPLICATION Smooth this over your face and relax for 15 to 20 minutes. Rinse off with cold water.

SKIN CARE DRY SKIN

In the same way you take vitamins, if you have dry skin, remember that your face needs them as well! Remember to wash your face every night before bed. In the morning, you don't need to use the cleanser; just splash your face with cold water.

SALTY DOG CLEANSER

1 cucumber

½ cup milk

½ teaspoon salt

PREPARATION In a blender, mix the ingredients together.

APPLICATION Pour a small amount of this onto a clean wet washcloth or sponge. Gently wash your face with this in the morning. Rinse with warm water.

SWEET BUTTER MOISTURIZER

1 tablespoon unsalted butter

1 teaspoon honey

PREPARATION In a small microwave-safe bowl, heat the butter for a few seconds to soften it. Add the honey and mix well.

APPLICATION Smooth this over your face in the morning and evening. Splash with warm water and pat dry.

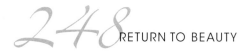

A MASK FIT FOR A KING

Aspirin promotes circulation, and the alpha hydroxy acid in red wine treats pigmentation.

1 tablespoon berries (strawberries, raspberries, or blueberries—whichever you like best)

2 teaspoons chopped fresh mint

1 baby aspirin tablet

1 tablespoon red wine

1 egg yolk

PREPARATION In a blender, combine the berries, mint, aspirin, and wine. Mix well, then add the egg yolk and mix well again.

APPLICATION Smooth this over your face and relax for 30 minutes. Wipe off with clean cotton balls; rinse with water. This is a very moisturizing treatment.

AFTER-DINNER MASK

1 teaspoon Cognac

3 tablespoons sour cream

½ teaspoon cornstarch

PREPARATION In a small bowl, mix the ingredients together.

APPLICATION Smooth this over your face and relax for 20 minutes. Wipe off with a soft tissue, then rinse with warm water.

THE BEST SHAVE

1. Boil several cups of water. Add a few drops of fresh lemon juice to the water.
2. Soak a clean towel in the hot water, then wring it out.
3. Use the towel as a hot compress on your face. Leave it on for several minutes.
4. After applying your shaving cream, begin to shave in the same direction as your hair growth. This keeps you from developing ingrown hairs.
5. Remember to apply aftershave.

SWEET 'N' CALM AFTERSHAVE

1 teaspoon dried chamomile

½ cinnamon stick

1 tablespoon vodka

PREPARATION In a small saucepan, bring 1 cup of water to a boil and add the dried chamomile and cinnamon stick. Turn off the heat, steep for 10 minutes, then strain. Mix the liquid with the vodka. Refrigerate in a clean plastic container.

APPLICATION Using a clean cotton ball, dab this over your face.

AFTER MOISTURIZER

3 vitamin E capsules

½ cup aloe vera gel

PREPARATION Cut off the tips of the capsules. In a small bowl, squeeze the oil into the aloe vera gel. Mix well.

APPLICATION Pat this over the shaved area, using a clean cotton ball, after you've applied your aftershave.

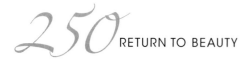

GREAT HAIR

SHINY HAIR MASK

1 teaspoon black tea

1 tablespoon castor oil

1 tablespoon almond oil

1 teaspoon vodka

PREPARATION Bring the dried black tea to a slow boil in 2 cups of water, then strain into a new pan. Simmer until thick. Over low heat, slowly add the oils. Add the vodka and mix well. Remove from the heat, cool, and refrigerate in a clean plastic container for 1 hour.

APPLICATION Cover your hair with the mixture and leave it on for 30 minutes. Use the time to shave, watch the news, enjoy your morning coffee—or just relax! Jump in the shower with your favorite shampoo. You only need to condition your hair lightly.

LAST BOTTLE OF BEER

If you have any left over from last night, use it on your hair! This is great for shine and makes the hair stay in place. And don't worry: the amount used is so small, it will quickly dissipate and won't smell.

Lean your head over the sink. Pour a few drops of beer over your hair. Massage it into your scalp, working toward the ends.

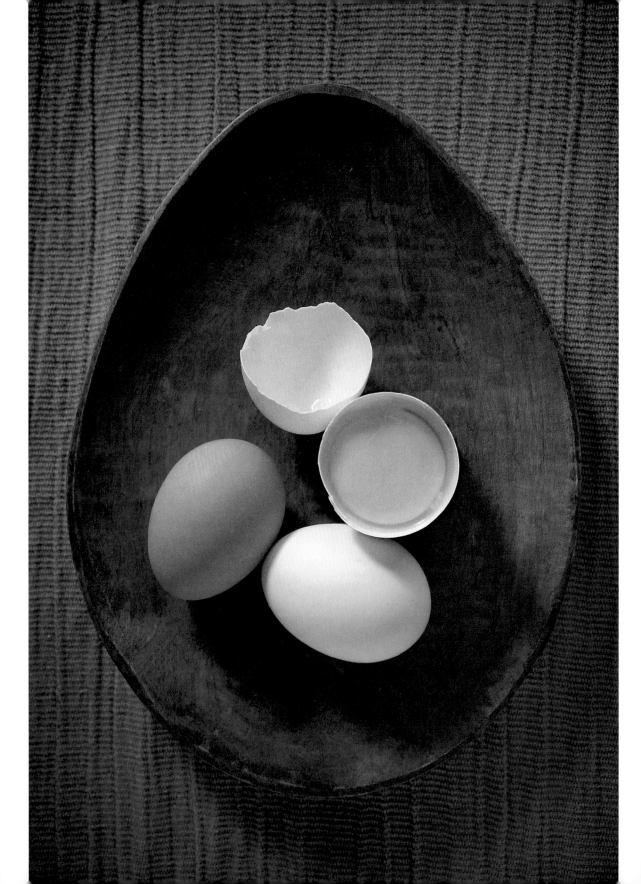

INDEX OF INGREDIENTS

BUTTER rejuvenates the skin and is an excellent moisturizer. 11, 35, 42, 66, 96, 137, 182, 195, 198, 248

BUTTERMILK has natural, gentle alpha hydroxy acid. 67, 133, 147

CABBAGE is rich in sulfur, copper, calcium, and vitamin C. Its leaves are soothing and have an anti-inflammatory effect. 22, 64, 151, 192, 207

CANTALOUPE is loaded with beta-carotene, high in vitamin C, and a good source of potassium and folate. 95

CARROTS contain all the great vitamins and minerals your skin needs to stay healthy and beautiful. They offer protection from the elements, and, as a bonus, their beta-carotene adds a hint of color to women with paler complexions—if used consistently. 18, 31, 60, 70, 79, 84, 161, 176, 192, 203, 204, 221, 235

CASTOR OIL is a deep moisturizer for dry skin and can be used for various skin irritations. 23, 199, 212, 251

CHAMOMILE contains an essential oil known as bisabolol, which has a number of anti-irritant, anti-inflammatory, and antimicrobial properties. 42, 59, 64, 120, 151, 161, 176, 177, 188, 195, 207, 215, 250

CHARDONNAY helps reduce wrinkles and fine lines by evening out skin tone and protecting against damage by free radicals. 184

CHERRIES are an antiaging fruit. They have been proven effective in fighting heart disease and inflammatory conditions. 121

CHOCOLATE helps to keep the skin clean and smooth. 204

CINNAMON is strongly stimulating to the skin and warms the body. 207, 250

COCOA BUTTER is a great emollient. It smoothes wrinkles and helps the thin skin around your eyes remain flexible and well moisturized. 12, 17, 47, 195, 204, 215, 233

COCONUT helps to remove age spots and acne scars. 149, 168

COCONUT JUICE (COCONUT MILK) strengthens and restores elasticity. 95, 116

COCONUT OIL/CREAM softens, protects, and promotes healing, and gives your skin a youthful appearance. 11, 34, 60, 71, 195

COFFEE GROUNDS can increase blood flow and circulation when rubbed on the skin. This is said to facilitate the breakdown of fats beneath the skin, eliminating cellulite. 153, 194, 247

COGNAC tightens pores and stimulates blood flow. 13, 121, 185, 249

CORN OIL soothes and softens. 94, 120, 177, 206, 207

CORNSTARCH calms and neutralizes redness in skin. 24, 30, 41, 53, 60, 132, 160, 181, 249

CORN SYRUP helps keep the skin hydrated and fresh. 42, 89

COTTAGE CHEESE contains amino acids, which help to bleach uneven skin tone. 13, 31, 61, 79, 89, 96, 152, 160, 161, 202, 211

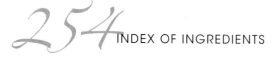

CRANBERRIES protect your skin from bacteria. Mildly acidic, they also offer gentle exfoliation. 66, 83, 128, 129

CREAM is a good base and a good moisturizer, and evens skin tone. 16, 34, 121

CUCUMBERS are hydrating and cause toning action in skin. 17, 29, 53, 60, 61, 88, 109, 136, 145, 203, 204, 211, 215, 218, 228, 236, 240, 248

DATES are high in fiber and potassium and prevent the skin from aging. 89

DILL has antibacterial properties and controls infection. It is also an excellent breath freshener and strengthens nails. 17, 190

EGG WHITES have tonic action and are best for normal-to-oily and oily skin. 34, 52, 61, 73, 79, 157, 164, 188, 190, 229

EGG YOLKS contain lecithin and are a natural emollient, which hydrates dry skin. 13, 37, 42, 53, 66, 90, 96, 116, 117, 121, 125, 128, 131, 136, 143, 148, 157, 161, 169, 176, 177, 178, 181, 184, 185, 186, 188, 194, 214, 215, 228, 247, 249

FIGS contain natural humectants—the perfect skin hydrator. 48, 112, 121

FISH OIL contains the omega-3 essential fatty acid that helps prevent wrinkles, slow the aging process, and maintain elasticity in the skin. 186

FLAXSEED OIL contains omega-3 fatty acids, which are highly beneficial to healthy skin. 83, 88, 112, 144

FLOUR reduces puffiness and redness of the skin. 16, 73, 76, 84, 102, 148, 178, 179, 188, 228, 229

GARLIC has healing benefits and natural antibacterial, antifungal, and antiviral properties. It also helps to treat acne scars. 206

GELATIN eliminates wrinkles and enhances the skin's elasticity. 30

GIN is a gentle, natural alcohol that closes pores. 95, 246

GRAPEFRUITS contain citric acid, which rejuvenates skin and closes pores. They also contain fructose and vitamins A, C, and D. Grapefruit juice is said to aid in collagen production, which supports healthy, smooth skin. 46, 76, 96, 148, 217

GRAPES are high in minerals and antioxidants. 40, 78

GREEK YOGURT not only binds ingredients, it hydrates, soothes, and gently exfoliates. 228

GREEN TEA is loaded with antioxidants, and it slows down the aging process. 210

HONEY is wonderful for older skin—it gently assists in sloughing away dead skin cells. 10, 12, 13, 24, 30, 36, 48, 58, 67, 72, 79, 82, 90, 96, 112, 116, 117, 121, 125, 132, 137, 144, 148, 149, 152, 153, 157, 160, 161, 164, 177, 178, 179, 181, 182, 184, 185, 186, 187, 189, 194, 199, 203, 204, 211, 214, 215, 219, 229, 230, 233, 234, 240, 247, 248

JASMINE is used externally to soothe dry and sensitive skin. 184

JOJOBA BEAN OIL helps reduce wrinkles and other signs of aging and also has antibacterial properties. 113

KIWI moisturizes and nourishes the skin. 94

LAVENDER is the perfect calming essential herb. 11, 145, 177, 203, 237

LEMONS are high in vitamin C. The citric acid closes the pores and helps skin maintain a healthy pH balance. 10, 11, 19, 30, 47, 54, 58, 72, 77, 96, 102, 109, 111, 112, 117, 131, 132, 136, 144, 157, 173, 188, 191, 207, 215, 218, 228, 232, 235, 246, 247, 250

LILY FLOWERS treat damaged and irritated tissue, rejuvenating skin. 11, 48

LIMES are overall one of the best rejuvenating foods for skin, and the juice prevents blackheads. 102, 120

MACADAMIA NUT OIL is a light emollient and is easily absorbed into the skin. 30, 190

MANGOES are high in vitamin C and antiaging beta-carotene, and leave skin feeling velvety soft. 35, 42, 54

MARGARINE is a natural humectant. 102

MAYONNAISE contains eggs, lemon, and oil—three great ingredients for skin renewal. It is also a good hair tonic. 36, 97, 109, 180, 187

MELONS are cooling and hydrating. They contain vitamins A, B, and C and natural sugars, which are healing for skin. 54, 137, 179, 217

MILK is a cooling, soothing, gentle skin softener. Lactic acid exfoliates dead skin cells—it's an instant skin beautifier. 14, 22, 28, 36, 37, 40, 46, 48, 52, 58, 59, 64, 70, 73, 82, 88, 94, 100, 111, 113, 116, 119, 120, 128, 132, 136, 149, 161, 165, 176, 177, 178, 179, 190, 191, 194, 206, 207, 214, 218, 236, 247

MINERAL WATER contains silica, which strengthens the cells between the collagen and elastin fibers. It also plumps the skin and slows the formation of wrinkles. Using sparkling mineral water is like giving yourself a mini spa facial. 10, 12, 29, 59, 70, 76, 95, 100, 148

MINT has a cooling, rejuvenating, and relaxing effect on skin. 23, 29, 41, 111, 113, 144, 192, 249

MUSTARD is good for preventing baldness and split ends and infuses shine into dull hair. It's also wonderful for alleviating bodily aches and pains. 145, 169, 191

NECTARINES make skin soft, smooth, healthy, and glowing. 73

OATMEAL contains an antioxidant called phytic acid, which soothes skin and is a gentle cleanser. 40, 42, 64, 72, 79, 82, 88, 100, 119, 144, 157, 176, 181, 194, 236

OLIVE OIL helps your skin retain its moisture, promotes a radiant complexion, and repairs sun damage. 10, 11, 19, 35, 40, 42, 59, 64, 76, 83, 84, 116, 120, 129, 151, 165, 176, 178, 184, 206, 214, 215, 228, 237, 240

ONIONS contain antioxidants, help to prevent acne, and stimulate circulation. 177, 206, 218, 229, 234

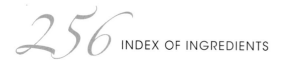

ORANGE JUICE is high in vitamin C, which helps produce a rosy complexion. 24, 70, 125, 132, 149, 153, 160, 168, 231

ORANGE ZEST (ORANGE PEEL) is a rich source of pectin and flavonoids. Pectin is a soluble fiber that scientists believe helps to lower cholesterol. Flavonoids are potent antioxidants. 47, 70, 149

PAPAYAS contain enzymes that literally digest dead skin cells. This fruit reduces age spots and fine lines and leaves skin feeling supple. 28, 66, 240

PARSLEY can reduce swelling and redness, lighten the skin, even skin tone, reduce blackheads, and aid in the prevention of wrinkles. 90, 132, 145, 210, 211, 214, 218, 231

PEACHES improve the complexion. Peach skin offers astringent action, which tightens the skin. 73

PEARS have abundant levels of vitamins C and K, which aid in healing bruises and lessening the appearance of dark circles. 14, 119, 168, 178

PEAS are a good food for blood circulation. They contain vitamins A and C. 49

PINEAPPLES are high in enzymes that remove dead skin cells; vitamins A, B, and C; and folic acid. 34, 65, 79, 199

PLUMS are a good source of antioxidant vitamins A and C. They also contain potassium and fiber. 89

POMEGRANATES contain more inflammation-fighting antioxidants than red wine or green tea does. When ingested, they are good for the lungs and relax the nervous system. They are also good for easing the effects of menopause. 28, 101, 160

POTATOES are packed with vitamin C—an antiaging miracle. Rich in potassium, potatoes soothe sunburn, acne, and dark puffy circles under the eyes. They also contain the mineral copper. Too little copper in your diet can reduce the skin's ability to heal, causing it to become rigid and lifeless. 23, 37, 109, 116, 127, 165, 179, 185, 207, 210, 212, 236

POTATO STARCH is an anti-inflammatory and has a natural drawing action that pulls toxins to the surface. 193

PUMPKINS are high in the mineral zinc as well as in beta-carotene, vitamin A, and vitamin C. They also contain antioxidants, which fight the free radicals believed to speed up skin's aging process. 22, 82, 83, 128, 144, 161, 210

RAISINS are high in iron. 117

RASPBERRIES are rich in vitamins A and C as well as in manganese. This fruit offers a calming and toning effect. 59, 234, 249

RED GRAPE JUICE is packed with antioxidants. 152

RED WINE helps to prevent the aging process and protects the skin from sunlight. 249

ROMAINE LETTUCE leaves are wonderful for oily skin. 120

ROSE OIL provides natural care for sunburn, wrinkles, and hyperpigmented tissue. 84, 145, 161, 194, 202, 228

ROSE PETALS calm and soften skin, adding a blush to your cheeks. 58, 77, 100, 229

ROSEMARY is used for binding loose, sagging, and hanging skin and is especially good for sensitive skin. 186

SAFFRON has antibacterial properties that make skin look brighter. 129

SALT is a great scrub for normal-to-oily and oily skin. 35, 40, 46, 52, 70, 82, 88, 101, 129, 145, 169, 199, 207, 210, 236, 247

SESAME OIL is a gentle emollient, safe to use during pregnancy. 133, 186, 233

SOUR CREAM lightens dark under-eye circles and is a wonderful skin softener. 10, 18, 23, 34, 47, 54, 79, 84, 85, 89, 101, 117, 129, 131, 143, 176, 180, 186, 199, 202, 203, 204, 215, 218, 230, 240, 247, 249

SPINACH is great for oily skin and minimizes pores. 191

STRAWBERRIES are packed with vitamin C. They also contain salicylic acid, which removes dead skin cells. 67, 76, 148, 164, 177, 234, 249

SUGAR gently sloughs away dead skin. 12, 61, 144, 157

SUNFLOWER OIL is rich in essential fatty acids. Its light texture is easily absorbed into the skin. 13, 41, 48, 54, 113, 117, 149

SUNFLOWER SEEDS are an excellent source of vitamin E, which is a powerful antioxidant. 78

SWEET POTATOES contain vitamin A (in the form of beta-carotene) as well as vitamin C, plus effective antioxidants for skin protection. 25

TANGERINES are rich in vitamin C. With strong antioxidants, this fruit refreshes and reenergizes your skin. 84, 101

TOMATOES have a natural exfoliating acid that removes the first layer of dead skin. They are high in vitamin C and lycopene, which helps reduce sun damage. 41, 53, 206, 240

TONIC WATER cools and tones. 246

VEGETABLE OIL is a great moisturizer for dry skin. 24, 89, 96, 180, 189

VITAMIN C tablets are the perfect anti-inflammatory. 65

VITAMIN E is easily absorbed by the skin. Rich in oils, it helps to reduce the appearance of fine lines and wrinkles. Its antioxidant activity fights free radicals, which come from pollution and ultraviolet light. 12, 43, 47, 71, 103, 199, 204, 233, 250

VODKA is a gentle antiseptic that helps to tighten pores. 29, 42, 47, 59, 71, 77, 101, 117, 131, 136, 168, 190, 206, 215, 231, 232, 250, 251

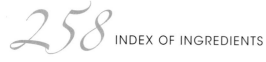

WALNUTS are packed with beta-carotene and vitamin E as well as a healthy dose of alpha-linolenic acid, which helps skin stay soft, smooth, and supple. 72, 112, 117, 129

WATERMELONS are rich in vitamins A, B, and C, and hydrate the skin. 41, 71

WHEAT BREAD is high in protein. It makes the skin care recipes nourishing and soothing and gives sensitive or dry skin a gentle exfoliation. 191, 218

WHITE BEANS contain calcium, potassium, and folate. 19

WHITE RICE lightens and brightens skin. 235

WINE VINEGAR is known for its high acid content and is used to remove alkaline residues from the skin. It also promotes blood circulation. 218

WITCH HAZEL restores acidity to the skin and fights off blackheads. 11, 17, 28, 41, 53, 71, 95, 168, 199, 215, 234

YOGURT provides a natural base for any recipe. It is a great skin softener and evens skin tone. 11, 17, 18, 24, 29, 30, 35, 42, 46, 49, 52, 60, 65, 66, 72, 73, 84, 94, 96, 102, 109, 117, 128, 132, 141, 153, 168, 177, 181, 184, 187, 188, 190, 203, 204, 237, 240, 246

ZUCCHINI is a good source of vitamins A, B_6, C, E, and K and is high in all the necessary minerals. 179

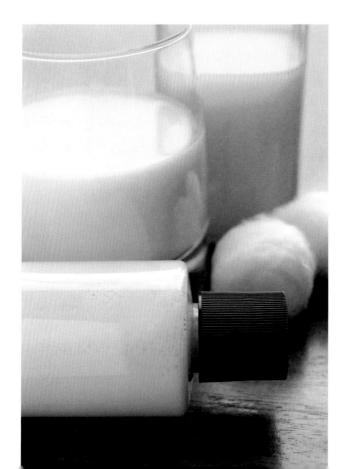

ACKNOWLEDGMENTS

From seemingly barren soil, spring blossoms.

It was April 2006. I was flying home from a job in Manhattan. The gentleman seated next to me struck up a conversation. Being a Gemini, I was only too happy to oblige him. He told me how lovely New York was during the spring and I told him how happy I was to go back home to see my son. Then he asked what I did for a living. "I help people bring out their real beauty," I said.

After I shared that potato slices placed under the eyes can eliminate puffy dark circles as well as a couple of other natural recipes, he proclaimed that he worked in publishing and that I had to write a book. I dismissed his idea with a laugh. The plane landed, and the passengers headed to baggage claim. Outside, at the curb, I felt a hand on my shoulder and turned around. "Write that book," the traveler repeated, and he walked away. The seed had been planted.

For several months, I thought about what kind of beauty book I would want to create if given the opportunity. Skin care isn't just my job—it has always been my passion. As a young woman, I trained in nursing, with a concentration in dermatology, in Armenia. When I moved to the United States, I opened my own salon. A few years later, I sold that successful business and happily joined forces with the team at Ole Henriksen Face and Body on Sunset Boulevard in Los Angeles. For the past thirteen years I've had the pleasure of treating some of the most beautiful and famous faces in the world, including Ellen DeGeneres, Prince, Jessica Alba, Carmen Electra, Charlize Theron, Bryce Howard, Alfre Woodard, and Kiefer Sutherland. My expertise, I realized, could benefit many readers.

One night shortly after finishing my book proposal, I attended Prince's publishing party. That evening I was introduced to the publisher of Atria Books, Judith Curr.

Judith handed me her card. "I'll be in Australia, but e-mail me. I'll contact you when I get back."

It didn't seem as if it should be that easy. I waited a week before I e-mailed her my proposal. The idea was to create a skin care book that looked as delicious as a cookbook. It would be filled with my fresh and easy recipes that women (and men) could make in their own kitchens. I wanted readers to fall in love with their faces. Judith e-mailed back an hour later, "I'm running out to the store to get cottage cheese for the mask." Suddenly, I was writing my book.

So here it is, my traveling companion, Hamilton, wherever you are. The seed grew and grew until it blossomed—juicy, ripe, and delicious. Thank you for your angel's whisper from the mouth of heaven.

I would also like to thank Ole Henrikson for inviting me into his world, Ruth Arzate, Judith Curr, and my editor, Johanna Castillo at Atria Books. Thanks to Justin Wheeler for his beautiful, delicious photographs, and to my fellow Geminis for their creativity and wisdom: Staci Greason, Robin McDonald, Svetlana Brezhnev, and little Jaquline. Much gratitude to my family for their patience while I worked on the book, and last, a special thank-you to my teacher, my grandmother Ermonia, for guarding the wisdom and stories of real beauty and passing them on to me, so that I might pass them on to you.

ABOUT THE AUTHOR

Before moving to the United States, Narine Nikogosian trained in nursing with a concentration in dermatology in her native Armenia and Russia. Narine's love of skin care was born early. As a little girl she would beg to go with her mother and grandmother to the local salon where they received facials. She began to experiment with whatever foods were in her mother's kitchen (vegetables, fruits, grains, and dairy), creating various concoctions that she would try on her own face. As she grew older, Narine combined the Armenian love of astrology with her love for skin care, producing successful recipes based upon the seasons, sun signs, and skin types; then she would invite her friends over to experiment with her treatments on them.

After moving to the United States, Narine opened and ran her own salon. Thirteen years ago, she sold her successful business to join forces with the team at Ole Henriksen Face and Body on Sunset Boulevard in Los Angeles. Private clients who receive Narine's specialized facials and take-home recipe instructions include Ellen DeGeneres, Prince, Jessica Alba, Carmen Electra, Charlize Theron, Bryce Howard, Alfre Woodard, and Kiefer Sutherland.